HEAL YOUR INNER CHILD

The Definitive Guide to Overcoming Past Trauma

and Developing Meaningful Relationships

with Time-Tested Therapeutic Techniques

Maria Clarke

TABLE OF CONTENTS

—

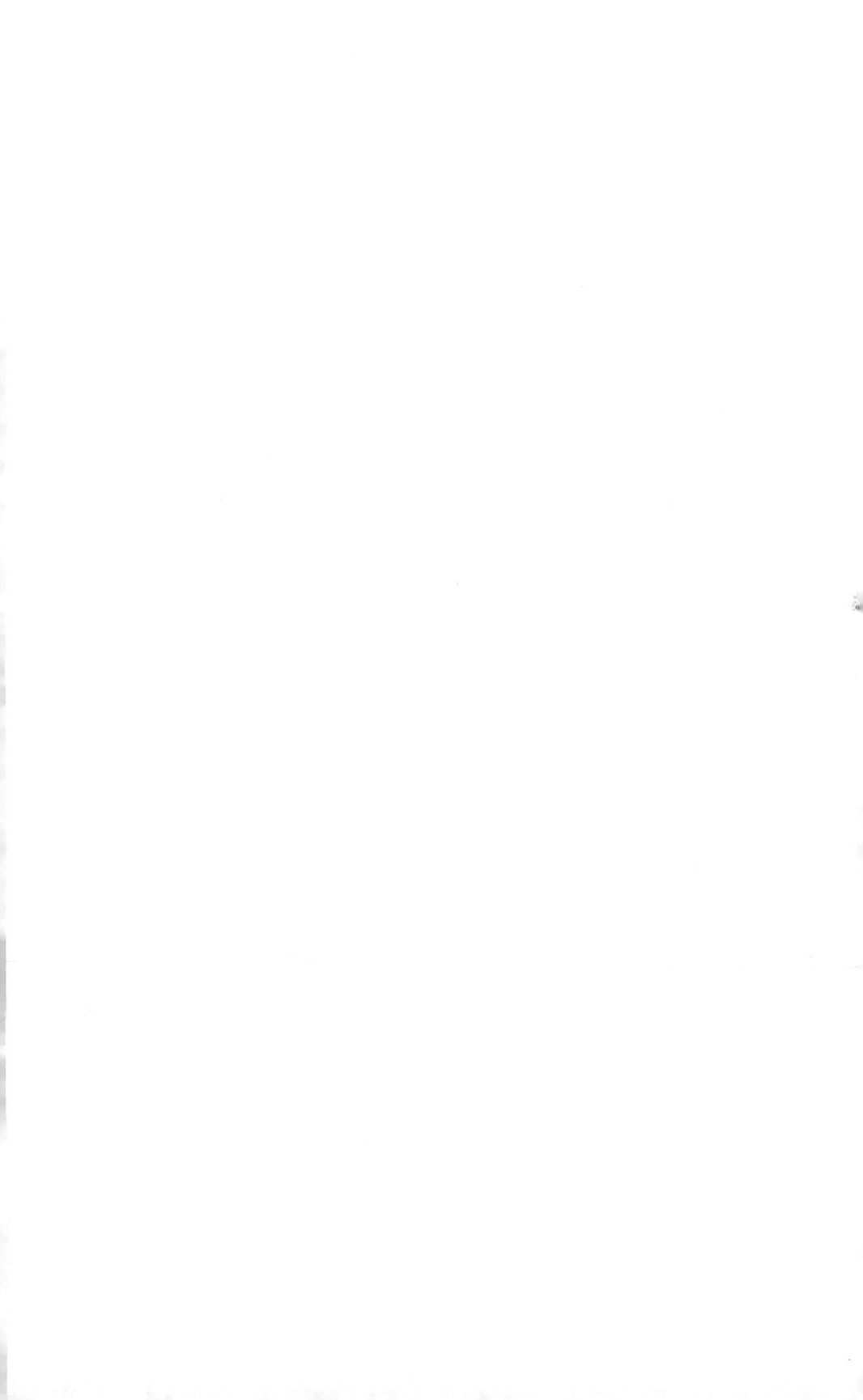

Dear readers,

I invite you to scan this QR code **using your phone's camera, aim at the code, then click on the link that appears** to access your bonus content:

SCAN TO CLAIM YOUR BONUS

OR

ENTER THIS URL IN YOUR WEB BROWSER:

transformationreads.com/bundle

(only use lowercase letters)

I sincerely hope this addition enhances your reading experience and aids you in your journey of healing your wounded inner child. Thank you for choosing to share this transformative experience with me.

Happy reading and listening!

Maria Clarke

'I don't want to be at the mercy of my emotions. I want to use them, to enjoy them, and to dominate them.'

Oscar Wilde

INTRODUCTION

——

In the tapestry of our lives, woven intricately with threads of joy, pain, and growth, lies a profound and often overlooked aspect of our being—the inner child. Our inner child represents the essence of who we were in our formative years, the innocent and vulnerable part of ourselves that experienced the world with wonder and curiosity. It embodies our innate needs for love, acceptance, and nurturing and holds the memories and emotions that have shaped our lives.

The inner child, for many people, is a happy and playful piece of themselves that they fondly recall from time to time—or all the time, if one is lucky enough to be that carefree. But for many of us, our inner child plays alone, and recollections of childhood memories only remind us of the heartache and trauma we were ill-equipped to deal with and still are to this day.

When you look back on your childhood, you may have memories that are shrouded in pain, anger, fear, anxiety, or a feeling of unfulfillment.

Oftentimes, it is easier to push these memories to the back of your mind rather than deal with the trauma they caused.

By submerging these feelings and not allowing yourself to acknowledge the damage they did to your emotional or mental state, you are stunting your ability to grow as a healthy adult. These emotions you have held inside since childhood can climb to the surface, distress your relationships, and affect your mental and physical health. This is why the combined use of this book's concrete exercises, advanced techniques and Dialectical Behavior Therapy (DBT) would help you overcome past trauma, manage your emotions and improve your relationships.

The concept of the inner child holds within it a profound sense of hope and possibility. It reminds us that the experiences and relationships we encounter in our formative years shape the very core of our being. Like a seed harboring the immense potential for a majestic oak, our inner child is a reservoir brimming with the essence of our true self, our authentic nature. It embodies our deepest desires, dreams, and boundless creativity. Yet, when the tender innocence of our inner child is wounded by the weight of childhood trauma, neglect, or unmet emotional needs, it can give rise to emotional turmoil, dysfunctional patterns, and a disconnection from our inherent truth. However, even in the midst of such struggles, there is a glimmer of hope, for the journey of healing our wounded inner child holds the promise of reclaiming our essence and embracing a future filled with transformation and wholeness.

We all carry with us an inner child who never goes away. Swiss psychologist and psychoanalyst Carl Jung said, "In every adult, there lurks a child—an eternal child, something that is always becoming, is never completed, and calls for unceasing care, attention, and education. That is part of the personality which wants to develop and become whole" (LibQuotes, n.d.). Your inner child may be the representation of your younger self or a fondness for the struggles and triumphs you overcame as your life spanned from adolescence to adulthood.

If you experienced trauma, neglect, or emotional pain that was too complicated for you to deal with when you were younger, your inner child is likely vulnerable and crouched in the corner waiting for someone to lead them to the light. Even though the pain of childhood devastated you and still does, you may feel that a rugged outer appearance is the only thing that is protecting you and your inner child from further pain.

Though we may tend to think that shutting everyone out will help protect us. In reality, it only leads to further seclusion and a lack of the compassion and love that we crave. Healing yourself from childhood trauma takes time, but it can be done. You only need to begin. Healing the child within will let them know you can take over and help protect them now.

I grew up in a family that lacked boundaries, and I was raised by strict parents who made me responsible for raising my siblings. I didn't get to experience childhood. Instead, I had to be mindful of everyone else and was not allowed to emote feelings of sadness or discontent with the role my parents decided to give me. I had to acknowledge, after years of struggling with my mental health, that I had grown up feeling repressed and unhappy.

Not everyone who has a wounded inner child considers their childhood overtly traumatizing, and many consider themselves lucky to have wonderful parents and come from a solid background. It is easy for most people to attribute early childhood experiences to whom they have become but be unable to identify any substantial events that could trigger negative events in present relationships. To identify what we might have missed in our childhood, whether it be attention or compassion, we need to divert from the narrative of good and bad and delve into what our past circumstances might have lent to what we feel was missing. You may not even realize you have a wounded inner child until you react to a relatively benign situation in a catastrophic way. The inability to respond to an adult situation appropriately may be your sign to look deeper into your past.

Before you begin a journey of healing, you need to acknowledge your inner child and get to know them by exploring your relationship. It isn't easy to identify your childhood as a traumatic one, but the only way to begin healing is to examine the past. Often, it is difficult to acknowledge a wounded inner child, but it can also come as a surprise to find out that you have one to begin with.

You may wonder:

- If I didn't have a super traumatic childhood, why is it important for me to work on my wounded inner child?

  Working on your inner child isn't about hating your family or placing blame but to identify any needs from your childhood that weren't fulfilled or pain that was inflicted upon you that has yet to heal. Inner child work is about finding the places in your life that need extra attending and then allowing yourself to respond. There is nothing in inner child work that demands you distance from or put blame on family or others from your childhood.

  Inner child work empowers people to act as their own parent. It allows you to give yourself what you need moving forward to ensure that any past neglect or pain is tended.

- What is the importance of identifying whether you had a traumatic childhood?

  There may be certain aspects of your life that have never connected the way they should, when everything aligns but a problem remains unresolved or you are unable to find happiness despite truly believing you have it all. When there are unresolved issues in your life that don't match your intentions or efforts, you need to determine if this is from childhood trauma. Issues can include

  - difficulty communicating with others

- having a hard time maintaining social and intimate relationships

- not understanding why your words or actions offend or hurt others

- feeling out of place, even within your own family

- being seen by others in a way very different from the way you perceive yourself

- How do you actually know if you need to work on your wounded inner child?

  If you are reading this book, you have had something happen to you that feels irreparable, or you know someone who has. You are traumatized by events that occurred in childhood and react to adult situations in a childlike manner. A wounded inner child presents differently for everyone, but for you, it may look like the following:

  - You subconsciously sabotage relationships.

  - You tend to attract toxic relationships.

  - You expect the worst from everyone.

  - You have difficulty saying "no" to people.

  - You cannot do anything right in any scenario.

If any of these sound like you, there is a wounded inner child who needs attention. Healing your wounded inner child can begin now that you are ready to acknowledge them and begin the healing.

'When we honor our inner child's feelings, we release the emotional hurts that we're still subconsciously carrying around.'

Patricia Hope

CHAPTER ONE

—

Signs you have a wounded inner child

W hether you have yet to acknowledge it or have always held their hand, you have an inner child who has shadowed or walked alongside you throughout your life.

Your inner child is a part of you throughout your entire life. They develop your personality and direct how you treat and react to others. It is the part of you that knows all your feelings, memories, desires, moods, and attitudes you have toward yourself. It is also a part of who you become as an adult based on how you were treated and the confidence and advantages you were given growing up.

Your inner child is the one who remembers the tune of a song but perhaps not the words and overcomes you with a feeling of warmth. Perhaps an aroma pierces your senses and allows you to visualize a much younger you cuddled on your father's lap on a chilly fall evening, or you reminisce about a warm summer evening with echoes of laughter. But not all memories of the inner child are welcomed.

Some people have an inner child who suffered at the hands of those who should have protected them, who neglected them when they should have showered them with praise, or who spoke words that their developing minds couldn't understand but felt the pain of just the same.

During childhood, people develop whom they will become, for better or worse, and navigate how to treat others and respond to various situations. For whatever reason, you may not have acknowledged your inner child; therefore, you may still carry the malformations of the past and the struggles and insecurities that come with it. If you break a bone, you do not leave it splintered. You go to the hospital and have it set. The same should be done with the fragments of your younger self that were never healed but need the proper attention to function in a healthy manner.

Some may not want to acknowledge their inner child, believing it to be a foolish ideology, but this is entirely untrue. Some people may be open to discovering their inner child, but not everyone believes they need to pay special attention to it. This regard could be due to an emotionally healthy childhood or having set the inner child aside for so long they feel a sense of normalcy. Take time to reflect on whether or not you need to give yourself the attention you always deserved by allowing yourself to revisit the vulnerable space you were in as a child.

Signs You Have a Wounded Inner Child

If you have always felt displaced but are not sure why, there could be unhealed wounds and deep-seated issues you are not aware of. To determine the mental state of your inner child, ask yourself the following questions:

- Did you feel safe as a child?

- Were you given freedom to express yourself?

- Did you feel you had a place within your family?

- Do you feel resentment toward people or instances from your childhood?

- How do you treat your inner child today?

Acknowledging and healing a part of you that has been broken or missing since childhood is a brave and important step in the emotional and mental healing you will go through now.

Your inner child not only lives inside your mind, but it is a part of your entire identity, inbred in your psyche. Staying connected to this part of yourself is what allows you to feel excited about upcoming events, drives you toward your goals and dreams, and determines how you feel toward others' success as well.

Connecting to the needs of your inner child that were not tended will help you overcome any emotional and developmental stunting you experienced because your psychological needs were not satisfied while your mind was developing. The insecurities you had as a child, along with the trauma you may have endured, carry on throughout your life because you are the child that you carry within you.

The child does not simply disappear as you age, just as your childhood isn't erased as you grow older. Sure, it may be more difficult to recall specific details from your early memories, but they are still there, living in the same mind you have today. You may have grown, and your experiences may be different now, but everything is connected to whom you were from the moment you were born.

What Does a Wounded Inner Child Look Like?

The wounded inner child carries the psychological imprint of your childhood traumas, the part of you that wasn't able to deal with what you endured when you were young. The part of yourself that was never heard and never healed is what you carry as part of your wounded past and the part of yourself that now acts as a protector by guarding the hurt part of you.

Several traumatic events or actions may have occurred to make your inner child need protection from yourself today, things that still make you feel vulnerable and unable to face these circumstances of your past. Life-altering events that cause extreme trauma may include

- loss of someone close to you, such as a parent, especially as a result of violent death

- losing your home to fire or poverty

- living through war or migrating to a new country

- going through a natural disaster like an earthquake or hurricane

Some recurring and equally psychologically damaging events can happen repeatedly throughout your life and leaves you traumatized, like

- emotional neglect from a parent

- stepping in as a caregiver when you were a child yourself

- dealing with the cruelty and ridicule of being a minority or having a physical disability

- being bullied for being different, like the way you dress or because you don't conform to societal standards

- dealing with prolonged neglect or rejection

People often feel they are not allowed to express their feelings when their distress does not meet extreme standards. You may feel your trauma isn't that bad by comparison to others, but pain doesn't have a limit. Just because someone else suffered the loss of a loved one doesn't mean that you need to hold in the disappointment of losing a job, having to move to a city far away from your family, or any other personal losses or disruptions. Your pain is as valid as anyone else's and should not be compared.

All of these can lead to an inability to have meaningful relationships with others. The feelings of being discarded or mocked can make it difficult to trust anyone, including friends. They may cause you to act with unwarranted negatively toward a friend or companion. This childhood neglect can also make you believe that poor treatment and half-truths are all you deserve, so that is what you accept or even look for in relationships.

The part of you, the child, that faced these painful situations wants to revisit these events, so you finally decide you can't move forward without acknowledging and healing the child you tried to leave behind. However, the protective part of you wants to shelter you from the pain you once faced.

Sometimes the part of you that is protecting your inner child does so by avoiding relationships entirely or by fearing commitment or intimacy and may find that pushing people away is the best defense.

Without facing the past and the pain that was inflicted upon you, you will never move beyond that stage of your life and learn to trust and love enough to have truly meaningful relationships. You may also find that success comes more easily to someone who has torn up their past, studied it, and rebuilt it with heartache but also with less self-doubt.

How the Inner Child Manifests

The inner child can manifest in several ways. Once you become aware of these manifestations of emotions and behaviors, you can identify where they stem from and begin to heal.

Low Self-Esteem

Low self-esteem can have many causes that stem from early childhood traumas, including feeling like an outsider with peers or at home, dealing with illness, or having a negative outlook of yourself despite self-inflicted expectations.

This negative way of viewing yourself often results in self-deprivation and a lack of self-worth, which can lead you to believe you have no value and deserve all of the negative aspects of your life. Additionally, a negative view of yourself can perpetuate anxiety and depression and can create issues with body image that lead to eating disorders.

To readjust your continual self-doubt, you need to acknowledge the struggles your inner child had to face and pull those memories and feelings to the surface. Loving your inner child and validating their emotions and feelings by way of self-parenting is the only way to move forward with a healthier view of yourself.

You Bend Over Backward for Others

People with unresolved trauma may find that they vie for the approval of others and will do nearly anything for attention. They may also put up with a great deal of mistreatment from someone during the course of a relationship, only to have it ended by the other person. This could be because of the fear to disappoint others or cause frustration, validating your worth by someone else's approval.

The part of you that will do anything to please others has likely been with you since you were young. You likely felt the need to keep your thoughts, emotions, and opinions to yourself because you knew it would cause discomfort in your home.

Your Boundaries Are Severe or Non-Existent

Often, a wounded inner child will manifest in how you interact with others, such as placing severe boundaries on relationships or having a complete lack of boundaries.

Many who suffer from a wounded inner child may not know how to set healthy boundaries with people. This can be evident by not being able to say "no" to others, even if it means you will be setting your own needs aside. This nagging persistence to please others may be due to not being able to set healthy boundaries with your parents as a child because you were afraid to disappoint them or make them mad.

It is not uncommon for parents to imply that by suppressing your own needs, you were being *good* by allowing your parents to set your needs aside. This can commonly arise in situations as an adult. You may feel that if you put your own needs first, others will be upset with you and dismiss you from their lives, even in intimate situations.

Alternatively, your boundaries may be rigid for self-preservation. This can result in distancing yourself from others who have offended you or hurt your feelings or cutting them out of your life entirely. There is no negotiation for resolution, and you move on without them.

You Withhold Emotions

Shame has no place in a child's life, yet many parents tell their children that expressing themselves in a moment of sadness or weakness is something to hide. As an adult, you may still hold that feeling, that expressing how you feel is a sign of weakness and something to be ashamed of.

There is no honor in shaming a child; it instills negative emotions and feelings of inadequacy, regret, or being unworthy of love. This can lead to severe emotions that manifest by way of treating others with disregard and bullying them to manifest the same emotion of *weakness* in them.

When a child is not allowed to feel their emotions without some placement of guilt or ridicule, they carry the feeling of shame that should be carried in a handbag by the adult in the situation, because they have been conditioned to feel they are the one who is *wrong* or *bad*. When a child acts out, this is often a sign they are repressed at home and unable to release feelings of pain in a safe, healthy, and completely normal way with a nurturing parent.

Fear of Abandonment

Particularly if you have experienced neglect or indifference shown to you as a child, you can have a fear of abandonment in adulthood that manifests by way of being insecure, clingy, and codependent in relationships.

Fear of being abandoned is one of the most damaging and common fears when you have had a traumatic childhood. It can give you a sense of insecurity in all relationships and you may act in an unhealthy or possessive way.

Trust Issues

Distrust is a common defense mechanism to avoid dealing with emotional pain, fears, disappointment, and anxiety. It often begins during childhood in someone who learned early on that they couldn't trust people, usually from an adult betraying their trust.

If you are already insecure about your abilities or your worth, trust issues become complicated. If you were gaslighted, made to feel worthless, neglected, or emotionally abused when you were young, building a sense of self is difficult and believing in your worth is even harder.

Being told you did not live up to your potential or you should have known better, would have seeded deep doubt and shame in your adolescent mind. It is difficult to trust others when you are carrying that psychological damage around.

Avoidance of Others

Many people who are described as introverts have a wounded inner child. You may avoid large social gatherings and only begrudgingly attend smaller get-togethers out of obligation. Perhaps you even get meals and groceries delivered to your house because being in public makes you feel overwhelmed. This is all common for someone who was not made to feel secure as a child.

Prone to Addiction

If you have easily fallen into an addiction of any kind, such as smoking, drinking, gambling, or other obsessive traits, it could be due to your childhood and the trauma you went through.

Addiction can be a symptom of an underlying and unresolved issue. Rather than dealing with the traumas and reliving the pain of them, you might block out what actually happened and welcome the rush of adrenaline as you overindulge.

Wounded Inner Child Archetypes

An archetype, as defined in Webster's Dictionary, is "the original pattern or model of which all things of the same type are representations or copies: PROTOTYPE" (Mirriam-Webster, n.d.). In simpler terms, it is a common representative of a specific person or thing. An example would be, "The movie was a good archetype of the horror genre."

In psychology, an archetype is defined as "an inherited idea or mode of thought in the psychology of Carl Gustav Jung that is derived from the experience of the race and is present in the unconscious of an individual" (Mirriam-Webster, n.d.).

According to Dr. Jung, the wounded child is one of the many child archetypes. Many believe that all people have all sub-archetypes to a degree and claim such things as all children have enjoyed magic or fantasy, not wanting to grow up, feeling left out, or fearing the dark.

The wounded child archetype is much greater in some people than in others and can be identified by the following characteristics:

- The person's behavior and characteristics can manifest in various patterns.

- The person can exhibit a fear of change and find comfort and reassurance in stability because they feel they are in control, which is something they never had in childhood.

- They likely have low self-esteem and feel worthless because they were undervalued in their formative years.

- They often feel their actions and words are misinterpreted or misunderstood by others, especially by those who have not gone through similar traumas in childhood and cannot relate.

- They are likely to suffer from clinical depression, anxiety, social phobias, and other psychological disorders.

- These people may find it near impossible to let go of emotional pain, both from their traumatic childhood and any new negative encounters they face as an adult.

- They can suffer from several pain disorders like fibromyalgia.

The above characteristics allow the wounded inner child to have empathy for others who may be going through a difficult time. They tend to feel drawn or closer to people who have had similar traumas in their own childhood and often try to help heal others, even before they learn to deal with their own feelings.

Often, those who have gone through difficult childhoods and have emotional and psychological issues, go through what is known as cognitive behavioral therapy to help determine the root cause of disruptive thought patterns and behaviors.

If you have a wounded inner child, it is easy to get caught up in a story of hopelessness, suffering, and gloom. There may be a constant theme of failure, rejection, feelings of worthlessness, and fear in the archetype of the wounded inner child. The wounded child likely feels misunderstood, unloved, abandoned, neglected, and forgotten, so much so that they forget to care for themselves.

Your inner child has unique wounds to be addressed, and the process of healing your inner child will be different from anyone else's since your home, the people you were raised by, and your circumstances were something only you experienced. Even someone who grew up with siblings can have a very different childhood or respond to situations differently because everyone's interpretation of experiences is different.

There are several wounded child archetypes. You may present one or more of the following:

- **The overachiever:** This archetype has a sense of value and acknowledgment through its success. They use validation from others as a coping mechanism for low self-esteem and self-worth, and they will only feel loved through their achievements.

- **The underachiever:** They keep to themselves and are often afraid to fulfill their potential for fear of being criticized or shamed for any potential failures. This archetype is afraid to become emotionally involved with others for fear of rejection, so they often avoid trying. They feel the safest hiding, as a wallflower, for no one to see.

- **The caretaker:** They are usually products of a codependent upbringing and have a sense of purpose and identity by neglecting that they need to care for others. This archetype is under the delusion that they will only be loved if they validate and care for others while neglecting themselves and their own needs.

- **The protector:** As a way of healing personal vulnerabilities, usually in childhood, this archetype is relentless in their pursuit of helping and healing others. They see others as incapable, helpless, and dependent and feel loved and validated for being in control of someone else's safety and happiness. They think they will only be loved by helping solve the problems of others and focusing on their troubles.

- **Life of the party:** These are the ever-cheerful and happy people who mask their pain, vulnerabilities, and weakness in a shroud of jokes and laughter. This inner child archetype feels their emotional state is shameful and the way for them to be loved and accepted is through making those around them laugh and be happy.

- **Idol-worshiper:** This inner child believes that love toward them is received by dismissing their own needs and modeling their lives after someone they admire. This is likely from a child who was hurt by the caretaker they worshiped and perceived as flawless.

- **Yes-person:** This person will dismiss their own plans and needs on a dime to help out others. They were likely raised by someone who gave plenty of themselves to others and was engaged in a codependent relationship or pattern. Their sense of self-value and feeling of being loved comes from being selfless and unflawed.

Inner child archetypes share the common theme that they are all products of neglected emotional needs and broken trust and connections. The roles they have adopted were used as survival modes to survive in a difficult upbringing. The narrative of the wounded inner child archetype was assumed subconsciously to survive at the hand of neglectful or demanding role models or people. These narratives follow the inner child throughout their lives, and they adapt to other relationships in a similar pattern without thought or predetermined ideals.

Archetypes are not accepted willingly. You assign this persona to all relationships throughout your life. The way to break free of these archetypes and strive for the person you are deep inside is to acknowledge that your inner child deserves to be heard for whom they were born to be.

Until you acknowledge the child deep within yourself, the wounded archetypes will demand to be heard and will create unnecessary drama or manipulate you into reevaluating your worth. Unprocessed trauma spawns coping mechanisms to protect against additional suffering.

What Is Cognitive Behavioral Therapy?

Cognitive behavioral therapy (CBT) is a well-known type of talk therapy whereby the affected person speaks to a therapist or psychotherapist over several well-structured sessions. Cognitive behavioral therapy helps form clarity of negative and skewed thinking so that unfavorable or challenging situations become clear and can be dealt with effectively by changing the way you respond.

CBT is especially useful for those who are struggling with mental health issues such as

- depression
- anxiety
- eating disorders
- phobias
- post-traumatic stress disorder

Unlike some talk therapy treatments, CBT helps deal with problems you are facing now. It helps you find useful and practical avenues to feel more positive about daily life by changing your outlook. Cognitive behavioral therapy helps you gain perspective on issues in your life that seem enormous and too difficult or massive to handle. Various techniques are used during CBT, such as

- coping skills
- stress management
- relaxation exercises
- learning how thoughts affect actions
- becoming more confident

Certain feelings, actions, and thoughts contribute to keeping you in a cycle of negativity or reliving situations that make you feel bad about yourself. CBT helps prevent the cycle of negative thoughts by dissecting what makes you feel anxious or frightened. When your problems are broken down, they can be managed more easily. This form of therapy helps you transform your negative pattern of thoughts into positive ones, changing how you feel. Unlike other therapies, CBT helps you deal with these issues over a specific number of sessions, not over several months or years like other talk therapies.

How CBT Can Help Heal a Wounded Inner Child

Trauma-informed cognitive behavioral therapy is focused on problem-solving skills that help change your physical and emotional reactions when you are confronted by something that triggers a childhood event. This therapy creates a safe place for anyone dealing with a wounded inner child with the hopes that they will feel safe enough to open up and begin healing.

The main goals of trauma-based cognitive behavioral therapy include

- reduced panic response
- increased trust and control
- effective and healthy responses to situations

The National Association of Cognitive-Behavioral Therapists says there are benefits to CBT and stated the following sentence, "Cognitive-behavioral therapy focuses on the idea that our thoughts cause our feelings and behaviors, not external things, like people, situations, and events. The benefit of this fact is that we can change the way we think to feel/act better even if the situation does not change" (Riopel, 2019).

The benefits of CBT in healing the wounded inner child can be

- anger management
- relapse avoidance
- chronic pain management
- dealing with negative emotions or thoughts
- dealing with sleep disorders
- building coping mechanisms for loss
- recovery from traumatic events
- dealing with relationships

With CBT, you are able to address and recognize what causes triggers and how and why destructive patterns become a part of your life. Once these negative aspects are addressed, you can replace the negative response with a positive reaction.

Connecting With Your Inner Child Worksheet

Several psychological modules describe the inner child as childlike, not childish. The essence of the inner child is that of being

- joyful
- sensitive
- curious
- playful
- innocent
- awe-inspired

Psychosynthesis, psychology of the self, calls the core of the child one's true self. This part of a person remains embedded in the subconsciousness of us all to make up our complete structure as a person. It is the part that craves attention, love, approval, acceptance, affirmation, and tending.

Answer the questions below to help you become more aware of and in tune with your wounded inner child by highlighting the behaviors you may be holding onto in your adult life, such as self-sabotage, dysfunctional behaviors, or attachment issues.

Ask yourself the following questions and answer honestly:

I frequently have trouble identifying my feelings.	yes/no
I find it difficult to express myself.	yes/no
I have trouble beginning things.	yes/no
I have difficulty following through with or competing things.	yes/no
I do not know who I really am.	yes/no
I often find my mind has wandered off and I'm daydreaming.	yes/no
I become anxious when I am in a new situation.	yes/no
I have trouble focusing on most tasks.	yes/no
I am fearful of the unknown and startle easily.	yes/no
I have difficulty saying "no" to people.	yes/no
I do not often go to social events on my own.	yes/no
I get nervous or afraid of going to new places.	yes/no
I feel horrible or guilty when I tell someone "no."	yes/no
I can't get rid of material objects. I hoard things.	yes/no
I do not feel that I am good enough.	yes/no
I am self-critical much of the time.	yes/no
I often wish I were someone else.	yes/no
I feel worthless.	yes/no
I am not a good person.	yes/no
I am an addict.	yes/no

I don't fit in anywhere.	yes/no
I feel alone in a room filled with people.	yes/no
I have trouble letting go of situations, anger, and pain.	yes/no
I am a very compulsive person and make impulsive decisions.	yes/no
I am always angry, and my actions tend to be aggressive.	yes/no
I feel defensive most of the time.	yes/no
I tend to avoid events and people.	yes/no
I usually eat too little or binge eat.	yes/no
I do not trust others.	yes/no
I avoid conflict.	yes/no
I am always nervous.	yes/no
I am rebellious.	yes/no
I do not ask for help.	yes/no
I am unable to stand up for myself.	yes/no
I have no close friends.	yes/no
I find intimacy in relationships to be very difficult.	yes/no

'To take care of ourselves, we must go back to take good care of the wounded child inside us.'

Thich Nhat Hanh

___

CHAPTER TWO

Healing Techniques for Your Inner Child

Now that you have met your inner child, it is time to listen to what they went through growing up. Give them a chance to tell you what happened to them by listening to what they had to say when no one else would.

In order to get any child to trust you, a connection must be made. To fully form a responsive and true connection with your inner child, release your inhibitions before beginning this process. There is no room for self-judgment when you are initiating the healing process of a part of yourself that has been judged and made to feel inadequate since childhood.

You can participate in many activities, such as art therapy, that will help you revisit your inner child.

The Importance of Creativity in Healing

Art therapy is a distinct method that embodies forms of expression via visual art as a form of psychotherapy. An entire profession is dedicated to helping people regain control of their emotions and relieve anxiety, but the great news is that you can benefit from this therapy by doing it yourself. If you doodle when you are nervous or use drawing as a form of emotional expression, then you are already applying the basic principles of art therapy to help calm yourself.

Creative healing is crucial to healing your inner child. Many think this is because children are naturally creative and express themselves honestly without questioning themselves or their abilities. Being creative allows an adult to become reacquainted with their inner child again.

As you age, you begin to lose passion for the simpler things, or you fall under the impression you are too old for such things. There is no original rule book that says to take yourself seriously once you hit a certain age. That was all assumed and enforced by society and it is contributing to a world full of suppressed and repressed adults.

Somewhere between childhood, where anything is possible, and adulthood, where you feel stuck in life and have no time for fun, your innocence and hope were lost. This can be especially true of those struggling with a wounded inner child, who never had the chance to experience a normal childhood. In an instant, your thoughts turn from what makes you happy to what society will think of your actions.

Over time, you stopped being yourself in front of others and only allowed your inner child to come out when nobody was watching. By the time your mid-teens came around, the inner child was repressed deep inside and neglected once again.

Reconnecting with your inner child will help you begin to heal from the trauma you endured. Let them know you still see them and accept them by engaging in art therapy and other childlike activities that will reignite that connection to innocence.

At some point during childhood, you lost sight of yourself and only looked through the eyes of others. Adults tend to develop an unhealthy obsession with having to be perfect, not to themselves, but to the perception of others. With art therapy, judgment and expectations need to be checked at the door so you can experience joy as you did before you realized others could judge you.

Art Therapy Techniques for Exploring and Expressing

Therapy is done by someone who is trained and licensed in that specific field, just as a psychologist would be licensed. Art therapy combines the process of creating art with psychological aspects and the past experiences of the person to help address areas of concern like emotional anguish. As mentioned above, this is not something you need to do professionally or pay any money for at all, unless you decide to do so later on.

Just as putting emotions into music, people tend to spill what they are feeling into their doodles, drawings, or even through lines. Art is a quiet way of loudly declaring through brush strokes, colors, and images how we are feeling on the inside. Trained therapists can use these visualizations to determine how you are feeling.

Art, in any form, is a form of self-discovery. There are, in fact, several types of creative therapies, including

- drama

- dance

- music

- writing

- visual expression

The process of making art gives you a sense of control over your own actions and can restore a sense of confidence to help you regain control of your life. Creating art therapy can include an expression of

- drawing

- painting

- finger painting

- carving

- molding clay

- sculpting

- making a collage

- doodling

When you undergo art therapy, you may be surprised by the feelings that emerge. Having a registered therapist direct these sessions can give you a better understanding of how to deal with the surprising responses and emotions that arise.

From the art, you and your therapist can interpret and discuss the work and go into the colors, images, and even the people included in the art, or those left out, to determine if this has a deeper meaning. Below are some examples of art therapy you can try:

Scribbling With Closed Eyes

As scribbling is a universal experience from childhood, it serves as a natural starting point for art therapy. Before beginning this activity, try to take a few moments to relax by engaging in a brief meditation or listening to soothing music. This exercise requires a few sheets of paper, some tape, and any writing utensils. Let's assume you're using colored pens.

Secure the sheet of paper to the table or surface you're working on with tape to keep it from moving. Next, select any colored pen of your choosing and position it in the center of the paper. Now, close your eyes and let the scribbling commence!

Scribble for approximately 30 seconds, then open your eyes. Observe your drawing closely and search for an identifiable image, such as a distinct shape, figure, or object. Take the time to examine your artwork from various angles. You may even want to hang it on a wall and step back to view it in its entirety. Once you have identified an image within the scribble, color it and add details to clarify it. Finally, hang your completed drawing and contemplate a suitable title for it.

Allowing yourself to scribble freely without constraints or expectations creates a space for subconscious thoughts and feelings to emerge onto the paper. Scribbling can tap into deeper layers of the psyche, accessing hidden emotions and experiences related to past traumas. By naming the image from your scribble, you assign a feeling or memory to it. Ultimately, this can aid you in reflecting and coming to terms with your childhood trauma.

Self-Soothing Image Book

Utilizing images can serve as a means of self-soothing and generating positive sensations. This exercise requires glue, scissors, collage materials, colored paper, magazines, and several sheets of paper.

To begin, reflect on any pleasant sensory experiences, such as tastes, textures, scents, sounds, and anything else that evokes a feeling of happiness or tranquility, and note them. Then, cut out images from magazines and other collage materials that align with these experiences.

Next, glue these images onto the paper, organizing them based on textures, composition, environment, or other categories. Finally, gather all the papers, create a cover, and decide how you would like to bind your book, such as placing them in plastic filing pockets and putting those in a binder.

After completing the visual aspect of the book, take a moment to write down your overall thoughts and feelings. Specifically, reflect on the emotions you experienced while selecting the images. Ask yourself questions like "Which sensory images did I prefer over others?" and "How are these images connected to my childhood experiences?" Then, feel free to continue adding to your book whenever you feel inclined to do so.

Spontaneous Image Journal

Engaging in regular image-making offers numerous opportunities for self-exploration and self-expression. By keeping and maintaining a spontaneous images journal, you go beyond simply pasting or creating images by providing a title and writing a few phrases or sentences about each piece of artwork.

To ensure that you can review and analyze your artwork and notes in the future, including a date for each entry is essential. By consistently using your journal, you can observe recurring themes, colors, and shapes in your artwork when you look back at your entries. This allows you to develop your distinctive approach to working with materials and creating your unique images and symbols. With time, your spontaneous images journal becomes a valuable resource for understanding yourself and your artistic journey.

How Does This Piece Relate to Your Other Art Pieces?

Experiment with images interacting with images. Create an additional artwork that responds to your original piece. Notably, the meanings attributed to your images may vary depending on the day or your current state. Remain open-minded and continue exploring the artistic process as a means of personal growth and self-discovery.

Which Parts of Your Art Do You Like and Dislike?

Choose an element within your artwork that captures your attention or evokes strong emotions. Then, immerse yourself in the creative process of producing a separate drawing or painting centered exclusively on that selected section. Next, expand its size, allowing room for additional details or imagery that emerge in your mind.

What Is Your Art Saying?

Imagine if the image could speak to you; what would it say? Assign a voice to each part of your artwork, allowing them to express themselves. Embrace a first-person perspective, allowing elements like a wave in your collage to communicate emotions by saying, "I am a wave, and I feel..."

What Emotions Does Your Art Convey?

Rather than focusing solely on the literal interpretation of an image, consider the emotions it conveys. First, reflect on your initial impressions and discern whether the image evokes anxiety, sadness, anger, happiness, or a combination of various feelings expressed through color, line, and form. Then, explore how you utilize shape, line, and color to convey and express emotions.

This therapeutic healing technique can reveal emotions and thoughts that have been buried for years. With a combination of your inner feeling being unveiled in your art and having a registered professional to help you talk through and acknowledge your pain, this can be a very effective form of therapy, especially for those who have unsuccessfully tried other forms of counseling.

Connecting to Your Inner Child

You may be open to finding and healing your inner child but not know where to begin. Here are some things you can do to connect in an organic way:

Maintain an open mind. Like with any new relationship, it may take you a while to get used to hanging out with your inner child. Begin by recognizing that your inner child is not only a part of you but that it is you. This child has a wealth of knowledge that you may have forgotten, things that are filed so far back in your mind that you can no longer recall, but they can.

You need not only to be able to laugh at the memories your inner child holds but also to dig deep into the recesses of your mind where dark memories are buried.

Revisiting your childhood can be a mixture of negative and positive emotions and events. All of the events helped shape who you are and gave you the means to make choices and reach your potential as an adult.

Be open to what your inner child has to say. Once you have made the decision to be open to meeting and getting to know your inner child, you need to listen without judgment to what they have to say. It is also imperative that you accept the feelings your inner child is expressing, no matter how difficult that may be.

You may learn that your inner child feels

- frustrated by ignored needs

- insecure
- shamed or guilty
- vulnerable
- abandoned or rejected
- anxious

Try to connect these feelings of inadequacy or sadness to a specific event that occurred in your childhood. This may help you identify what similar situations trigger you as an adult. For example, if your partner needs to go to work on the weekend instead of staying home with you and spending time together, disappointment and frustration can erupt. Your feelings of rejection may present in a way similar to that of a child's tantrum.

If you look at your reaction to this adult situation, you may be able to find a time in your childhood—or many times—when your parents couldn't spend time with you, had to cancel a special outing because they had work obligations, or traveled for work and their time for you was sporadic.

This insight may help you understand why you are reacting a certain way toward your partner when they cancel plans, and it may help you open up more direct and effective forms of communication with them.

Hearing what your inner child is saying and how it is feeling will allow you to go through those emotions again without trying to push them deep down. Acknowledging your feelings and giving them a place in your life can help validate your experiences and the distress they caused you. It is also an important step toward accepting that you have some things to work through.

Study children. There is much to be learned from watching your own children, the children of friends, or those of family members. Children are a great example of living in the moment and enjoying the slightest majesty in life. Find a memory from your childhood when you couldn't wait to be done with school or dinner so you could fall into your own imagination and mold into a princess, superhero, or some other fantastical imagining.

If you can, play hide and seek, skip rope or play tag, and see if it brings back the simpler times in your life. Play allows a child to express themselves, but adults can feel the freedom of youthful expression if they allow themselves to. I often find that reading a story from my youth helps bring back a time when I was able to escape from my own discipline, if only temporarily.

Pull out old photos and reminisce. Looking through old photos can help trigger childhood memories and emotions, some that you may have completely forgotten about. Talking to your parents or siblings and sharing old stories can help bring emotions to the surface that were buried deep down. While this may lead to some wonderful stories, it may also help you ascertain where some of your trauma comes from. Be prepared to deal with those feelings head-on.

Act like a child. People often scoff at those with childlike qualities, but acting like a child now and again is essential to your mental health.

If you were unable to enjoy your childhood because there was a lack of positive and fun experiences, you need to enjoy those aspects now. You might have missed out on getting ice cream on the beach or camping and roasting marshmallows by the fire as a kid, but you are still here and so is that child deep down.

Enjoying carefree experiences such as jumping in mud puddles or playing in the rain will help you reconnect with a part of yourself that was missing. If you have children, sharing these moments with them will not only give them a sense of a complete childhood but will also restore one to you.

See a therapist. Opening correspondence with your inner child can be a lot for anyone to handle on their own. Hiring a therapist can allow you to navigate your emotions in a safe place and can provide helpful tools for you to begin to heal your inner child.

Connecting with a therapist who deals with past trauma and the exploration of the inner child is crucial for your healing.

Psychodynamically oriented psychotherapy can help you get insight into the problems you are facing today, but it evaluates patterns people tend to develop over time as well. To identify these patterns, the therapist will ask for details during therapy sessions about

- thoughts
- emotions
- childhood experiences
- beliefs

By noting these patterns, the therapist can examine ways you avoid confrontations or stress or develop defense mechanisms to protect yourself. Once these patterns are identified, it is easier to learn strategies to cope with these avoidance tactics and begin to face your problems.

Leave room for wonder. Healing is a continual journey. By initiating a bond with your inner child, you are cultivating awareness for what this long-neglected child needs. You may also learn new details and wants that shouldn't be ignored.

Stay connected to the innocence of that child that never gave up wondering what it would be like to slay dragons or if they could climb a tree into the clouds. Reset your mind to be more open to speaking with your inner child on a regular basis. Be sure to listen when you feel a nudge of discontent and see what part of your past needs to be reconciled.

Allowing the relationship with your inner child to grow over the years and making them a part of who you are today will allow you to change and grow.

10 Questions to Awaken Your Inner Child

Maybe you have tried to stir your inner child in the past but have felt silly and decided it was better to return to adulting. Like most things, it takes time to get into the mindset of a child and to excite the wonder and adventure you used to feel before responsibility and time crunches took over your life.

If you have had a hard time finding that child who would run into the rain with an umbrella that would never be opened or the kid who went foraging to see how many beetles they could find, you may be going about it all wrong. No child is going to approach an adult who is sitting with their hands clasped and a sneer on their face. You have to pique the interest of the child within by reassuring them that you remember.

Here are some things to ask yourself to awaken your inner child:

- What did you want to be when you grew up?
- What was your favorite thing to do?
- What did you always wonder about when you were young?
- What were you prone to daydreaming about?
- What astonished you most as a child?
- What was your favorite thing to play with?
- What was your favorite subject in school?
- What was your favorite thing to make art with?
- When you are around children now, how do you feel?

Take the time to acknowledge what your inner child is saying without judgment or redirection. Connecting to your inner child means you are always open to listening, and you feel compelled to live your life the way that makes you feel free.

Connecting With Your Inner Child Worsheet

Now that you have connected to your inner child, staying in touch with your younger self is essential for proper healing. Take the time to enjoy activities that brought you joy when you were a child or that you never had the opportunity to do because you never had a proper childhood.

Read each goal below and write notes on how you are honoring your inner child by participating in these goals.

- I was open with my inner child by…

(Listen to what your inner child has to say. What did they say today?)

- Observe your inner child. What did you learn from them?

(Write a letter to your inner child.)

- Speak openly with your inner child.

(Write in a journal using your inner child's voice.)

- Watch children for guidance.

(Look through childhood photos and other mementos. What memories did they bring back?)

- Do activities you enjoyed as a child. What were they?

(How did you live at the moment?)

'To confront the pain of the past is to unlock the potential for a brighter future.'

Carl Jung

———

CHAPTER THREE

Exploring Inner Child Wounding

To better understand your inner child and where the hurt comes from, it is helpful to gain perspective on the innate qualities of children. All children are born with certain common traits, but the potential or quality of these traits is reliant upon how they are nurtured, ignored, or manipulated.

These inherent traits were described by John Bradshaw, author, counselor, and public speaker, in the acronym, WONDERFUL, as defined below:

Wonder

Children live in a state of natural wonder because they live in each moment without expectation of what comes next but with excitement to see what does. As we age, we lose this sense of awe and fall from our state of constant surprise into a sense of responsibility.

Optimism

A child is born with the unconditional belief that they can trust those around them and that goodness is constant. When adults who are responsible for that child's care become unpredictable, the trust fades and dissipates. In a way, the world is rose-colored for children. If, however, it becomes unhinged, their world can shatter and cause doubts and insecurities.

Naivete

The concept of limitations does not exist in a child. From the moment they are born, children explore whatever and wherever they can without fear, protected by their caregivers who set boundaries, instill a sense of safety, and teach about danger while supporting this unwavering need for independence. If the adult is not diligent or willing to provide the necessary boundaries and enforce them with patience, a child may be put in a dangerous situation or taken advantage of.

The opposite can be said for an adult who is overprotective of their child and doesn't allow them to explore the world, even within their guidance. If a child is sheltered, they may not be able to incorporate themselves into the real world when the time comes since they are not equipped with the tools or experiences to integrate into regular situations.

Dependence

A child is helpless and unable to survive on their own. They need to be cared for and taught how to transition from a loving and supportive environment into taking responsibility for themselves. Some caregivers don't want to relinquish their role and keep the child dependent on them, thereby stunting their own abilities to care for themselves.

Some adults can swing in the other direction and be neglectful of their child(ren) or expect too much of them. In this situation, a child may grow into an adult who isolates themselves from others or becomes overly dependent on a relationship with a friend or significant other.

Emotions

There is no shame in laughing at what delights you and crying when things make you sad. A child has no ability to deny themselves the feelings they have unless an adult steps in and tells them what they are feeling and how they are responding is not okay. This teaches the child to be ashamed of displaying emotions.

Resilience

The expression that kids are resilient is not an overstatement. Kids have the amazing ability to adapt to new environments and to move on from uncomfortable situations. They have no preconceived notion of what is to come, so they are able to accept their surroundings and situations at face value. It is when an adult places boundaries on a child's ability to move on that we see an issue arise.

Free play

Children are filled with wonder and spontaneity. They have a natural sense of wonder that compels them to imagine wonderful things that seem very real in their wondrous mind. In the beginning, there is play without a need for anything but fun. This changes when a child becomes older, and the focus shifts to winning and goals, rather than just enjoying free play.

Uniqueness

It is important for a child to feel they are special and unique as they are, that they are complete no matter what. At some point, as our identities form, there can be disapproval from others or expectations that cannot be met. A child needs to be accepted for all that they are, without being told to change to comply with the expectation of others.

Love

All people are born with the disposition to be loving and show affection. Children are compelled from birth to need their parents and to feel safe in the arms of someone they trust. Often, a struggling parent may respond to a child who is not behaving the way they want by telling them that they are bad or that they never listen or always do things wrong. It is important to use language that lets the child know they are not using appropriate behavior, but they should know it is not a reflection of them, and it does not make them bad.

Inner Child Wounding

Allow yourself to recognize your childhood for better or worse. Your childhood experiences affect the adult you are today. The two phases of childhood and adulthood are both a part of you and the experiences you went through. Often, people are reluctant to acknowledge that the emotional development and mental health issues they have as adults stem from their childhood.

Also known as *attachment wounds*, inner child wounds can derive from traumatic childhood experiences. The responsibility of creating a safe and supportive environment for a child is the responsibility of the child's parents, but this is unfortunately not always provided.

The inner wounds of a child are

- **Abandonment:** You may have a fear of being abandoned by loved ones or being left out if someone abandoned you when you were a child.

- **Trust:** You may be afraid of being hurt if you were not protected from harm by your parents or adults in your childhood.

- **Guilt:** You may have difficulty setting boundaries or asking for help as an adult because you were made to feel guilty when you were a child.

- **Neglect:** If you were neglected as a child, you may have repressed emotions, trouble saying no, or low self-esteem.

Inner Child Wounds

Abandonment:	Guilt:
• Feel left out • Fear of being left • Don't like being alone • Codependent • Tend to attract those who are emotionally unavailable • Threaten to leave	• Feelings of being sorry • Don't like to ask for help • Use guilt as manipulation tactic • Afraid to set boundaries • Usually attract people that make you feel guilty
Trust:	**Neglect:**
• Afraid of being hurt • Don't trust yourself • Don't feel safe • Look for ways to distrust others • Insecure and in need of external validation • Attract those who feel unsafe	• Low self-worth • Difficulty letting go • Angered easily • Repress emotions • Difficulty saying no • Afraid to be vulnerable • Tends to attract those who don't make you feel seen or don't appreciate you

Questions to Get to the Root of Healing

You may not know what you went through in your childhood to bring on feelings of self-doubt and pain. Ask yourself the below questions to resolve this issue, develop a greater understanding, and eventually heal your inner wound.

- Were you bullied as a child?

- Did you feel neglected as a child?

- Did you fit in at school?

- Do you feel your voice was heard?

- Did you feel safe growing up?

- Were you ignored?

- Did you have appropriate boundaries?

- Was there an instance where you felt like something was wrong with you?

- When was the first time you lost trust in someone?

How is Your Wound Manifesting in Daily Life?

It can be frustrating when you work hard to have good relationships and do well at your job, only to feel underappreciated and misunderstood on a constant basis. If you find that despite your best efforts, you are still falling short, it may be your inner child manifesting in your daily life.

When issues from childhood go unresolved, they get carried over into our adulthood in the way that we deal with situations and people. Our emotional scars carry over from childhood and affect our lives until we acknowledge and resolve them. It can be difficult to lead a fulfilling life with meaningful relationships when people perceive your behavior as untoward.

Moving forward, remember that the work you do will help heal your inner child and give you normalcy in life with stable relationships.

Effects of Childhood Trauma

Would you ever expect your five-year-old to make the meals, pay the bills, and run your errands? Of course not! This would be a tremendous and unrealistic expectation to put on a child. Those who have a wounded inner child are asking themselves to do the impossible and live a productive life that is essentially being run by the inner child.

In some adults, the wounded inner child can present itself with mental health issues and disorders. To function as a healthy adult, you need to work on healing your inner child so the behaviors you learned when you were young don't continue to run your life today.

In some cases, it is important to seek the help of a mental health professional to help you deal with trauma from your past, especially if it stems from a severe or life-changing event. Once you have worked through the bulk of your childlike behaviors, you can begin to implement behavioral strategies and implement productive behaviors.

Signs Your Inner Child is Running Your Life

Not everyone is able to determine if their lives are being interrupted by a still unsettled and hurt inner child. Once you are able to identify the following signs in yourself, you will become a step closer to appealing to your younger self and regaining control of your own decisions.

These are some signs that your inner child is the one in control:

- **Emotional versus logical thinking:** Often in life, we face the inevitable outcome of something not going as planned. In these circumstances, you may become angry or feel you were the victim, even plotted against. If your initial reaction stems from emotion rather than a logical perspective, this may be a sign that your reaction is coming from your inner child.

- **Difficulty assuming responsibility:** If you find it challenging to maintain the daily tasks you have committed to, or if you often bow out of your responsibilities, then your inner child may be doing the delegating. Responsible adults usually have no issue fulfilling their obligations. Even with reluctance, they still get it done.

- **Repetitive behavior:** You may notice similar patterns in relationships in your personal and work life. If this is the case, take note. These patterns might not be particularly harmful to anyone, but they should be addressed and recognized as a potential nudge that your inner child needs attention.

- **Substance abuse:** It is not uncommon for someone struggling with a wounded inner child to turn to drugs or alcohol to help them cope with their unresolved emotions. If you feel this is the only way to numb the emotional pain you are dealing with, this is a cry for help to listen to your inner child.

- **Legal troubles:** While getting a parking ticket or traffic violation once in a blue moon is common, you need to pay attention if you have a pile of unpaid tickets, arrests, or other legal issues stemming from a pattern of disregard for the law.

- **Instability in relationships:** If you have a pattern of disrespectful behavior from or toward others that leads to unstable and or unhealthy relationships, this is a strong sign that you have an inner child in need of proper care. Often, someone who has not healed their inner child, will cling to and often seek out unproductive or toxic relationships that they know will never last.

The Four Attachment Styles

Attachment styles vary among people and are how we interact with and bind ourselves to those with whom we are closest. Identifying and understanding your attachment style can help you in several ways.

The four attachment styles are

- Secure

- Anxious-preoccupied

- Dismissive-avoidant

- Fearful-avoidant

These attachment styles stem from childhood and play a part in our relationships when we are adults. They can determine the success or difficulty of our romantic lives, yet when issues arise, we don't link them to when we were younger.

What Do Attachment Labels Mean?

These attachment styles are primarily defined by our behaviors. For example, if someone is anxious about attachment, they could be clingy to their partner. An anxiously attached person may want to be in constant contact or close to the object of their affection at all times. It can be very stressful for that individual if they are separated from their attachment which can cause anxiety. They can even display sadness or anger when reunited with the person they are drawn to, which might serve to remind the person of their love or punish them for leaving in the first place.

Someone who has avoidance in attachment could show more cold or indifferent behavior. They may consider themselves to be independent, when they may be removing themselves from the possibility of engaging in healthy relationships. This person may even feel they should show their detachment from partners or family by placing a higher priority on work, hobbies, or others whom they barely know.

As children, people become attached to their parents or caregivers and put their unwavering trust in them to keep them safe. The quality of that guidance and care, or the lack thereof, then informs our attachment styles as adults. Romantic relationships are the ones that have particularly strong attachment styles since these are most akin to the earliest relationships we had with those who cared for us in terms of vulnerability and familiarity.

Attachment Styles in Relationships

Every adult attachment style has distinctive relationship elements. However, these are only generalizations and not certainties. Understanding these patterns can help determine how your attachment style can negatively or positively affect your relationships.

- **Secure attachment:** Those with this attachment style are able to maintain suitable boundaries while having intimate partnerships. These people go into their relationships confidently and have low anxiety about their associations. Those with a secure attachment usually communicate effectively on any given topic, including problematic ones. They have a positive outlook on their relationships and are forward about what they need and want in those relationships and expect their partner to be upfront. If these people are unattached, they are not bothered, since they are generally comfortable and happy to be on their own.

- **Anxious-preoccupied:** Those with the anxious-preoccupied attachment style tend to be apprehensive in their relationships and may need frequent affirmation from their partner. This can often lead someone with this type of attachment style to magnify or invent conflicts within their relationships because they get a sense of security when they focus on these issues. They are also more pessimistic about their relationship and have a more anxious and paranoid outlook on the connection they have with their partner. This may originate from fear of losing their companion, and they may act jealous or possessive.

- **Dismissive-avoidant:** People with the dismissive-avoidant attachment style may come across as distant or cold and may be cautious of entering into a committed relationship, often insisting they don't want to settle down or be tied to one partner. These people can show their dismissive-avoidant style and independence by focusing on hobbies, work, or socializing with acquaintances, while simultaneously leaving their romantic partners out of the plans. This type of person is likely to display narcissistic traits and be passive-aggressive.

- **Fearful-avoidant:** People with fearful-avoidant attachment styles tend to be drawn to toxic relationships. This may be a result of their desire for a meaningful relationship but also their fear of an intimate relationship. They may want to be close to someone but may feel too vulnerable for the commitment that comes with it. Those with fearful-avoidant attachment push their partner away while simultaneously obsessing over them by showing affection one day and ignoring them the next day. These people tend to have a difficult time setting healthy boundaries within relationships.

Self-Sabotage

You may see a pattern in your life where problems recur and prevent you from reaching your goals. Even after making changes and setting forth a path for success, you end up failing time and again. If you keep asking yourself why you can't overcome a hurdle or why failure chases you around, the answer may be very simple: You're self-sabotaging. This refers to behaviors or patterns of thought that prevent you from reaching your desired goals.

How to Stop Self-Sabotaging

As discussed, self-sabotage is likely to stem from a wounded inner child who has low self-esteem. Perhaps your parents, who weren't particularly successful in life, told you that you should focus on getting a job that would cover bills and nothing more. After all, who are you to go to a university and get a degree? If you were told from an early age that you weren't going to be successful in love, money, or life, then you may self-sabotage, because it makes you more comfortable to go without than it does to have what you want. You may even feel unsettled when your life is going well, because feelings of genuine happiness are disrupted by thoughts of what is inevitably (in your mind) going to go wrong because you certainly don't deserve a happy life.

Treatment to Help You Stop Sabotaging Yourself

Anyone who self-sabotages may find it challenging to regulate their behaviors and emotions. Emotional and behavioral dysregulation is frequently formed during childhood due to neglect or trauma. Harmful reactions can come from this dysregulation.

Fortunately, there is help for those who self-sabotage using various vices, such as

- excessive alcohol and drug use
- self-harm

- binge eating

- angry outbursts

The below therapy options, explained in further details in Chapter 5 of this book, are available to those who self-sabotage:

- **Cognitive behavioral therapy (CBT):** This form of therapy uses techniques effective in relieving cognitive contortions. These techniques help you change negative thought patterns into more positive solutions to help raise your well-being.

- **Dialectical behavior therapy (DBT):** This therapy is helpful for those who are dealing with intense emotions, mental illness, and even personality disorders. This therapy is a way to learn how to regulate and better understand your emotions.

Healing your inner child will allow you to see yourself as a whole person, rather than the fragmented individual you have held together thus far. There is more to life than mediocrity, and it begins when you allow yourself to accept that you were hurt as a child. Only once you learn to acknowledge this fact, will the healing truly begin.

'In acceptance, we find the power to transform our wounds into wisdom.'

Jack Canfield

———

CHAPTER FOUR

—

Embracing Your Inner Child Through Acceptance

It can be overwhelming to initialize the healing process of your inner child, especially when you didn't know there was any healing to be done. A big part of moving through the trauma and acknowledging and dealing with the hurt from your childhood is allowing yourself time to relax and be calm in between these momentous steps.

Especially where hurting is involved, we need to allow ourselves to accept who we are, practice healthy self-acceptance, and validate our past experiences and emotions. Relaxation techniques are a way to help manage stress and return your body and mind to a state of calm.

Stress can have long-term effects on your physical and mental health, so particularly in times of need, it is crucial to focus on reducing stress through relaxation techniques. There are numerous benefits from detangling your mind and entering a state of calm, including the following:

- slowing your heart rate

- controlling your breathing

- improving digestion

- lowering blood pressure

- stabilizing blood sugar

- reducing anxiety

- stabilizing stress hormones

- improving sleep quality

- reducing fatigue

- stabilizing mood

- improving mind clarity

- increasing problem-solving abilities

Relaxation Techniques

Professional therapists can help you integrate relaxation techniques into your life, but there are also many techniques you can do at home. Relaxation techniques require you to focus on something calm to help increase awareness of your body. Choose the type of technique that speaks to you the most and gives you optimal benefits.

You may want to try a few of these techniques before deciding on one or alternate throughout these relaxation exercises:

- **Progressive muscle relaxation:** With this technique for relation, you focus on tightening each muscle group and then relaxing them. This can help isolate and make you more aware of physical sensations when the muscles alternatively tense and relax.

  To begin, you can tighten the muscles in your feet, and then relax them. Continue to focus on isolating, flexing, and releasing the various muscle groups all the way up to your head.

  Try to find a peaceful area where there are no interruptions and at a time during your day when you can usually find calm. Flex your muscles for around 5 seconds, release for 30 seconds, and repeat.

- **Autogenic relaxation:** Autogenic means self-generated and refers to, in this case, using visual imagery and your own body awareness to lessen stress.

  For this relaxation technique, you visualize a peaceful place that calms you. Focus on your breathing becoming even and your heart rate slowing down, then relax each part of your body one by one until you melt into a relaxing state.

- **Visualization:** In this technique, you are going to use a mental image and visualize a place you love that makes you feel calm and safe and promotes a feeling of peace.

  Using visualization requires you to use as many of your senses as possible, such as sound, smell, sight, and touch. If you visualize a beach, imagine the wind on your face, the smell of the ocean, and the sound of the waves crashing on the shore.

  Sit in a quiet and comfortable location, close your eyes, and revisit your favorite place, focusing on your breathing while thinking happy thoughts and repeating positive affirmations.

Simple Relaxation Techniques

Some additional simple relaxation techniques to bring you some calm amid a hectic day include

- yoga

- deep breathing

- meditation

- massage

- tai chi

- aromatherapy

- music and art therapy

- hydrotherapy

Relaxation Techniques Take Practice

As you practice relaxation techniques, you will learn to be more in tune with the physical effects of stress, such as muscle tension. You can take a more active role in how your body responds to stress by providing an outlet when you begin to feel the symptoms come on. Utilizing these techniques can prevent stress from overtaking your life and can help prevent depression and anxiety.

Relaxation techniques take time to master so don't be hard on yourself or feel you have done it wrong if you don't feel much initial benefit. It will take time to master relaxation techniques, as it does with any other skill.

Try a few different relaxation techniques to see which is best for you. If one doesn't work, that might not mean that you failed at it, but that it wasn't the best way for you to destress.

The Healing Power of Acceptance

Your inner child has dealt with emotional neglect for years, so the best thing you can do is to acknowledge them. You have already taken a step toward showing them they are being heard and their pain is being validated.

Validation means to show someone you acknowledge their emotional journey. When you judge or ignore someone, the person feels they are being rejected and that their feelings don't matter.

You don't have to agree with the person's actions by validating their feelings. You are showing them that you understand their perspective on a situation, but are by no means suggesting you would do or feel the same way. Validating someone's feelings lets them know they are seen, no matter what your personal opinions on the matter are. You are simply acknowledging that they are accepted for who they are. This same message can be sent to our inner child.

By validating their experience and hearing their voice, you are letting them know that they are seen and heard.

Validating Your Inner Child's Experiences

Go back to the discovery of your core wounds. It is important to identify the wounding that occurred and what your inner child is holding on to so that you can validate their emotions.

You need to begin validating your inner child by being present and interested in what they dealt with in childhood. It may be difficult to articulate how they feel in the beginning, but be patient and allow them to work through their feelings in a safe place, without being rushed or judged.

The next step is to nurture their wounds by responding with words of affirmation and assuring them their feelings are valid and their reaction to their wound is understandable. Here are some examples of what to say to let your inner child know that you are listening:

- I see you and I hear you.

- That sounds like it was difficult to go through.

- It sounds like that is a lot to handle.

- That must have been really hard to deal with.

- I acknowledge your feelings.

- There is no such thing as a bad child.

- Your mistakes do not define you.

- I understand that must have been scary.

- Adults should never put that responsibility on a child.

Healing Exercises for Your Inner Child

Below are some healing exercises you can do to relieve your inner child:

- **Validate:** The first thing you need to do is validate the feelings of your inner child. Always begin with reassurance and empathy, and let them know that their feelings are valid. It is important to let them know what they feel is proportionate to what they went through. It is important to include this step and face your inner child with compassion and empathy and not simply force your way through this first stage.

  By validating your inner child, you are acknowledging the pain you went through in your childhood. As painful as it is, you need to associate the pain of your inner child with the initial link that it leads from your past and make sure you process those emotions.

When you identify these childhood traumas and acknowledge that as an adult, you still suffer from these wounds, you will be able to work through them and begin to move forward. By identifying the event from your childhood that led to the wound of your inner child, you will be able to move forward and let go of the painful past.

An example of validating your inner child would be

Of course, you feel afraid and alone right now. You were never made to feel safe because your parents would dismiss your fears, no matter what they were of. If you were afraid of the dark, they would tell you to go to bed and dismiss your fears. I am here and I am listening to what you have to say. I understand that you can be afraid and not understand why, and that's okay. I'll help you figure things out.

- **Separate:** Once you have emphasized with your inner child and validated their feelings, you need to make the distinction between right now and the past. Let your inner child know that they are whole and good, no matter what happens. Relay what happened to them was not because of who they are; the pain was not their fault. Use actual examples of differentiating between now and the past so the inner child believes they are safe and the things that hurt them in the past are really behind them.

An example of separating the past and present would be

You should not be ashamed of the fear you feel; that is something your parents taught you. Being made to feel ashamed of being afraid was wrong. I validate your feelings, and I am not going anywhere. You will not have to go through anything alone and feel unsupported as you were when you were a young child because I am here to protect you. It is my honor to reassure and support you. It is okay to feel scared at times, and I am happy to comfort you.

- **Have a positive vision:** Once you validate your inner child and differentiate, it is important to continue the dialogue with a positive vision that will bring a feeling of comfort, inspiration, safety, and freedom to your inner child. This can be a vision that becomes increasingly large over time into a more detailed vision. Once you have shared this vision, you should experience a sense of release, and you will feel light, calm, peaceful, and lucid.

An example of a positive vision would be

Now that we have found one another, we are going to be able to move forward in life with a greater sense of peace and closure every day. Let's go for a walk and just enjoy nature.

Choose Self-Compassion Over Shame

Shame is a terrible feeling to have and is unwarranted in most circumstances. This negative feeling is attributed to self-judgment over something we feel we should hide from other people. Practicing self-compassion is a way to be kind to yourself and diminish the feelings of shame that self-judgment magnifies.

Shame is usually ingrained in us from childhood because someone who was in charge of our happiness also implied that we were bad or had done something unforgivable. The thing with children is that they don't forget as easily as people assume they do. Moments that are damaging to emotional well-being can be a lifelong challenge.

It's not easy to overcome shame just because you can identify when it began. It often requires a lot of self-work, often with the guidance of a mental health professional.

Have Some Compassion for Yourself

Self-compassion, or lack thereof, is directly correlated to feelings of shame, anxiety, or embarrassment. Be kind to yourself, and you will find it comes more naturally as you deal with your past pain, emotional experience and the shame you were made to feel.

Pain and Emotions

There is no way to avoid negative experiences throughout our entire lives, but how we react to those situations can have a significant impact on our behavior. For example, if you react with shame to a negative experience, you are displaying self-criticism that can cause you to isolate yourself from others.

Your self-confidence and self-esteem can become extremely low when your inner voice is heckling you. Depression, drug use, eating disorders, and anxiety in social situations are also linked to low self-confidence. When you withdraw from people, you isolate yourself and make it unlikely that you will build or maintain a support network and meaningful relationships in your life. When you distance yourself from others, you are making your world, including your support network, very limited.

Causes for shame can include

- body image

- relationships

- work

- health

- sex

- religion

- money

- trauma

- being labeled

What Is Self-Compassion?

Self-compassion allows you to reassure yourself and calm your anxieties when you are going through times of doubt.

You may need to work on the skills to become self-compassionate, since it involves being able to accept yourself as you are and understand where your mental state and feelings are coming from and how to avoid self-judgment.

Examples of self-compassion would be saying to yourself things like the following:

- "Today I didn't do as much work as I wanted to. Tomorrow I'll get on it first thing."

- "I'm allowed to express what I am feeling, especially when someone is not respecting my boundaries."

- "If I want to spend the day at home reading, it doesn't mean I'm lazy; it means I'm taking care of myself."

Keep in mind that showing yourself compassion is not the same as making excuses. If you didn't do something you promised you would, own up to it, but if you set out to do more than you were capable of doing, all you have done is mismanaged your time. Accept you are not perfect—none of us are—and embrace the beauty of not expecting every little thing to go right.

Overcoming Shame

We know how damaging shame can be and that it affects our self-confidence and self-worth. It is crucial to override this toxic feeling to be more productive by accepting yourself as you are or changing the way you think about yourself.

Allowing yourself to be kinder to yourself and abolishing shame will help you shed the burden you have been carrying around with you. Shame is not conducive to a healthy relationship, especially with yourself. Give yourself a healthier outlook on life by initializing your self-worth, no matter what anyone else says or thinks.

Practice Visualization to Soothe Your Inner Child

Visualization is an effective way to connect with your inner child and help deal with childhood trauma. To use this method to help heal your inner child, create a safe place where you can connect. Visualize a place where you feel empowered and safe; somewhere you are away from critique. Once you are in your beautiful, visual garden, at the beach, or anywhere that you feel safe, invite your inner child to talk things through.

To begin visualization, do the following:

- Choose a quiet, calm area.

- Close your eyes, breathe deeply and purposely, and relax.

- Imagine you are walking down a serene, winding path. The path is your safe place where you feel supported and untouchable from anything harmful.

- Once you have found your safe place, take some time to allow the ambiance to seep into your core. Is it bright and colorful or dim and calming? Is there a creek rolling in the distance or wind blowing through the trees? What does it smell like?

- Once you have become acquainted with your safe place, picture your inner child walking down the same path toward you.

- When you greet your inner child, embrace them warmly and show them they are loved.

- Once you are both settled in, ask your inner child to tell you when they first felt shame, fear, or loneliness. Word it in a way a child would understand and respond to.

- Wait patiently for them to answer.

- Tell them you appreciate them and acknowledge their pain.

- Say your goodbyes and watch them leave.

- Walk back down the path and out of your safe space.

- Return to your conscious state.

Follow these basic steps, or something similar, to meet with, acknowledge, and release your inner child. This needs to be a confident place where emotions are allowed in all their forms.

Children see the world differently than adults, even our own inner children. You may assume certain events didn't play a part in your wounded inner child because you perceive those situations differently as an adult, but as a child, they might have been extremely painful. You can never assume on behalf of your inner child.

Through working on your inner child, you will learn to grieve, heal, and work through the trauma you have held subconsciously throughout your adult life. This can signify a release from the emotional barriers you had with your inner child and provide you with spiritual maturity, emotional balance, and well-being.

Prompts for Journaling to Connect to Your Inner Child

Part of validating your inner child is listening to what they have to say. Journaling is an important part of this journey and should be done often. If you are not sure how to begin a conversation with someone you know well but haven't spoken to in years, here are some prompts to get you started.

Ask yourself some of the following questions:

1. What did I enjoy playing most as a child?

2. Did I have a favorite place to spend time?

3. What was I happiest doing?

4. What made me feel safe and content?

5. What was something I missed out on as a child?

6. Did I get to be with friends? If not, why? If so, how did I feel when I was with them?

7. How can I make sure I experience what I lacked in childhood?

'With each reframed memory, we paint a brighter tomorrow.'

Pat Bluth

—

CHAPTER FIVE

Reframing the Past

As an adult, you have gone through experiences and have gained a perspective that impacts how you expect life to go. Some of the experiences may be uncomfortable to consider.

Often, enlisting the help of a therapist can be useful, especially if you are spiraling in a pattern of negative thoughts and emotions. When reframing is used in a therapeutic capacity, it is referred to as cognitive restructuring.

Reframing your past can be beneficial to your mental state. Mental reframing is when you shift your mindset to look at a specific person, relationship, or situation and see it from a marginally different perspective.

Cognitive Distortions

Cognitive distortions are predisposed outlooks we see in the world around us. These are illogical beliefs and thoughts that we reinforce over time.

These sequences can be subtle and challenging to recognize when they are a part of our every day. Since they are such a consistent part of our lives, it can be difficult to see that something needs restructuring.

Cognitive distortions can come in several forms but all share commonalities. The cognitive distortions are as follows:

- patterns of thinking or beliefs

- tendencies that are inaccurate or untrue

- the potential to inflict psychological harm

Admitting you have false beliefs and distorted thoughts may be terrifying, but no good comes from relieving these facilities daily.

Anyone can have cognitive distortions, even if only occasionally. Those who have consistent distortions struggle with identifying and modifying these incorrect ways of thinking.

What Is Cognitive Reframing or Cognitive Restructuring?

Cognitive reframing or restructuring is a restorative exercise that allows the client to challenge, replace, discover, or modify their defeatist thoughts or cognitive distortions. It helps people reform their false way of thinking about themselves and those around them. Therapists use this tool to reduce stress by encouraging more positive and productive thoughts.

It may seem unfathomable to change a negative mindset that has regurgitated through your mind for years, but just as with any other skill, it becomes easier to second-guess your disruptive thoughts over time.

Our thinking can make us believe in variations of the truth, which seems shocking, considering the majority of our thoughts are rational. These cognitive distortions are a biased way to think about our environment. They are beliefs and patterns of thought that are illogical, inaccurate, and false and have the ability to hurt our self-confidence and our ability to be successful.

Magnification or minimization is the most common cognitive misrepresentation. They affect how we gauge what goes on around us and to us.

Types of Cognitive Distortions

Below is a list of the most common cognitive distortions:

- **Polarization of thoughts:** This disorder occurs when a person creates acute thoughts surrounding polar opposite groups (something is good or evil) and ignores median steps with unrealistic proportions. A polarized thought is distorted and can cause great emotional distress.

  An example of polarized thinking would be to think in extremes, such as you are either going to find love or be alone for the rest of your life.

- **Selective filtration:** With this disorder, the one affected eliminates all positive events and deflects the attention onto the negative, augmenting them. The person takes comfort in the negative characteristics to interpret their actuality.

  Someone might only see their failures and consider their lives a mess without acknowledging the success in life. Those with this distortion revisit the scenarios in their life that they fear most.

- **Overgeneralization:** This means that one negative incident will become the normal ending for all other similar situations. In the event, if something unfavorable happens one day, the individual will likely think that the bad thing will happen every time. This can also be compared to the oppositional view that something will always be or never be a certain way.

- **Demand and perfectionism:** Inflexible and strict ideas of how other people and themselves ought to be. The person is always seeking satisfaction within themselves or others because they are finding something wrong in everything.

  The consequence of this is guilt, low self-esteem, and frustration with thinking they always fall short of expectations. Their unwavering demands on those around them cause others to feel anger toward them.

- **Projection:** The person displays frustration, weakness, or problems they don't want to acknowledge and expects others to have these characteristics too.

- **Elimination of the positive:** This thinking implies that people exclude the positive achievements in their lives by chalking it up to luck or chance or by saying positive events are rare events that don't frequently happen when they are oblivious to the majority of these good events.

- **Magnification and minimization (catastrophic vision):** Catastrophic vision is a distortion that can trigger anxiety. It is depicted by the person expecting that the worst-case scenario will always occur or that the situation is considered more serious than it is.

  Minimization represents the opposite thought in those with anxiety. Obsession or depression mainly consists of ignoring the good moments or events that occur in their lives. When you are unable to appreciate the good moments in your life, your happiness and quality of life suffers.

- **Personalization:** In this egocentric way of thinking, the person with this cognitive distortion thinks everything people say or do has something to do with them specifically and that the world revolves around them.

  These people tend to take everything personally, even when they have nothing to do with the situation or event. An example you might notice in yourself is taking responsibility for circumstances that were out of your control or not your fault. These people may also make the incorrect assumption that they were targeted or intentionally left out.

- **Emotional reasoning:** This is the inaccurate belief that the way you are feeling is what is real, that the way you feel within a situation is reality. Expressing your feelings and receiving validation for those feelings is important, but so is reacting to a situation based on facts and evidence.

- **Labeling:** This is a cognitive distortion where people reduce themselves or others to one characteristic that is likely negative, such as a loser or drunk. This labeling defines someone based on one act or single event that can cause the person to berate themselves and underestimate or misinterpret others.

Managing Distortions

Fortunately, there are ways to manage these distortions over time. Don't expect an instant remedy, but the following thoughtful changes can help change thought patterns, including:

- **Identify the thought.** Figuring out why you are having depressed or anxious thoughts is key to figuring out how to dissolve them. Understanding the depth of where these issues are rooted will allow you to dig them up and out of your subconscious.

- **Look for alternative thinking.** Look for variations to your thinking, such as alternative reasoning, positive interpretations, and objective evidence to elaborate your thinking. There is often another explanation you can come to when you put thought into it. Try writing your original thought on paper, and then write three alternative interpretations, and see where your thinking ends up.

- **Analyze the productivity of your thoughts.** When behavior provides some sort of positive response or benefit, people tend to repeat the action. Analyze how patterns in your thought process may have benefitted you and initiated coping mechanisms in the past. Do they allow you to feel in control when you otherwise would have felt powerless? Do they let you get away without admitting to taking risks that were unnecessary? What are the cons and pros of cognitive distortion and what does it take from you?

Cognitive distortions are habits in your thinking patterns that can be negatively biased and untrue. These distortions normally develop over months or years in response to negative events.

Cognitive Restructuring

How you perceive a situation affects the way you respond to it. Our responses and perceptions are strongly guided by feelings. If you have an inaccurate, exaggerated, or instant response or interpretation to an event in life, you may go on having distorted perspectives of reality, otherwise known as cognitive distortions.

Cognitive distortions not only shape your feelings and thoughts but also your behavior, and they can have an effect on your health, especially in the long term. By practicing cognitive restructuring, you are challenging your perspectives and thoughts. Practice techniques that will build fresh insights into an event or situation, and create a more balanced perspective.

Ask yourself the following questions to challenge your perspective:

- Is there evidence to back up my perspective?

- Is there a side to the situation that I am unaware of?

- Would others come to this same conclusion?

- Is there a gray area I'm not taking into consideration?

- Am I holding myself to unrealistic expectations?

- What is affected by my way of thinking?

It is common to become wrapped up in cognitive distortions, but recognizing them will allow you to take control and challenge them. Ask yourself questions to challenge the distortions, thereby creating a perspective that is more balanced.

Cognitive Restructuring Worksheet

Which behaviors did your caregivers use in your childhood?

- Blaming
- Teasing/laughing at
- Manipulating
- Physical or emotional withdrawal or abandonment
- Betraying
- Shaming
- Criticizing
- Patronizing
- Enmeshment

- Invalidating
- Conditional love

In what ways do you use them now?

Behavior ➡ Action

Think of the situations in which these things happened. What would have been a nurturing response?

Situation ➡ Nurturing Response

Examine the Evidence

Socrates was one of the most influential philosophers in history. He died in 399 BC. He stressed the importance of reflecting on our thoughts by exclaiming, "An unexamined life is not worth living" (Reference, 2020).

Socratic questioning is an effective tool for contemplation and promoting problem-solving and self-discovery. This can be a constructive catalyst for managing mental health issues such as depression and anxiety. In Cognitive behavioral therapy (CBT), the client and therapist work together to search for the logic behind negative thoughts and irrational beliefs.

Therapists often use Socratic questioning when they want to help the patient confront the distorted ideas they have and gain more mental clarity and emotional and behavioral stability.

Socratic Questioning in CBT

Socratic questioning encourages you to ask questions that promote self-reflection and initiate problem-solving. It is often used in CBT to help with the assisted discovery process.

It works with the collaborative philosophy practiced in CBT which includes working with a registered therapist to identify and help replace negative thinking patterns. This has become known as a favorable approach to therapy to help improve the outcome for patients by enabling them to explore various perspectives, which leads to a new way of thinking and more validation in feelings and clear thinking.

Why Is a Question Considered Socratic?

This type of questioning helps you explore something in greater depth, identify relationships, and form greater clarity in your thinking.

The qualities that make a question Socratic are below:

- **Clear:** Questions must be direct and free of unnecessary ramblings. A Socratic question is straightforward and clear; easy to understand.

  An example of a clear Socratic question is, "Why do I always feel bad about myself after I hang out with Charlotte?"

  An example of a more ambiguous question that could have many answers is, "Why am I always like this?"

  This unclear question can have many answers, because the specific behavior isn't named. To analyze properly, the actions, people, and situations all need to be set out clearly.

- **Open:** To encourage discussions and produce more helpful thoughts, ask open-ended questions. Open-ended questions lead to answers that require more thought and then to have a more detailed explanation. They can also be less intimidating and increase the opportunity to have a more fruitful dialogue.

Open-ended questions are ones that cannot be answered with a simple "yes" or "no." To keep a conversation going and to get adequate information, you want to ask questions that are open, such as the following:

- ○ Why did you decide to go into nursing?

- ○ What is the most jarring experience you have gone through?

- ○ How do you imagine your life in ten years?

- **Neutral:** Neutrality is important, because if you ask a biased question like, "What's wrong with me?" then you are already assuming an answer and therefore are not acknowledging reality. By avoiding biased opinions, even by yourself, this type of question becomes powerful, because it provides unlimited possibilities and not just the perception you have at the moment.

- **Focused:** Specific questions can open up new avenues of learning and drive us to delve into new topics and discover new things. The question needs to be on a specific topic or issue. By examining one particular problem, the Socratic question can bring us a greater understanding of our thinking.

Examples of Socratic Questioning

The following are examples of Socratic questions:

- What did you mean when you said…?

- What is the point of…?

- Give me an example.

- Do you mean…?

- What did you expect the outcome to be?

- Are there different points of view? What is an example?

- What was the most important thing about that question?

Finding a New Perspective

Cognitive distortions can be changed over time, and a new perspective can be found. Here are some steps that you can take to help change your way of thinking and have more productive thoughts:

- **Identify the thought causing you anxiety.** There are going to be specific thoughts that make you feel anxious or cause you to feel depressed. The first step is to recognize what that thought is and the responsible distorted thinking.

- **Reevaluate the situation.** There is always a gray area or alternate explanation for what has occurred. Try implementing objectivity and look for a more positive interpretation of the situation that you deemed negative. Things are not always what they appear to be.

- **Evaluate your gains.** As difficult as it is to admit, you may be perpetuating negative behavior because it brings you an outcome that benefits you or gives you a feeling of accomplishment. Ask yourself the following questions:

  - Are you behaving in a way that gives you a feeling of superiority?

  - Do you feel in control of the situation when you interpret a scenario or situation a certain way?

- Does your behavior allow you to avoid taking responsibility for something you have done?

Determine how your thought patterns have affected relationships, jobs, and other connections you may have lost. Considering what you are missing out on might allow you to take control of your unhinged thoughts.

Cognitive behavioral therapy

Cognitive behavioral therapy (CBT), as we have discussed, is a form of therapy that helps someone identify and interpret descriptive ways of thinking and change them to a more healthy and optimistic pattern.

This form of therapy allows you to focus on what you want for yourself in the future and helps you set goals to get there. You can look forward to a more stable relationship with yourself and others within a few weeks to months as results become apparent.

Socratic Questioning Worksheet

Those who are suffering from a wounded inner child or other neurological or mental illness are likely to have an inner dialogue that never shuts off. The mind can conjure up thoughts and scenarios that provoke a negative response or emotion and affect the way we perceive and respond to a situation.

To prevent your rampant thoughts from running your emotions, take the time to respond to each thought by questioning whether the emotions it is making you feel hold validity. Some examples of the questions you could ask yourself would be:

- Is there evidence supporting the thought? Disproving it?

- Is the thought based on feelings or on facts?

- Could I be making assumptions and misinterpreting the evidence or situation?

- Is this a black-and-white thought that I am having or the more complicated reality?

- Could others interpret the same situation differently? What are those interpretations?

- Am I considering all the evidence or just looking for ways to justify my perception of the situation?

- Are my thoughts an exaggeration of reality?

- Did this information come from someone else, or did I witness this?

- Is my thinking the worst-case scenario, or is it a likely depiction of the truth?

- Is this a thought I usually have, or is there a specific fact that supports it?

Reparenting and self healing

You have introduced yourself to your inner child, accepted them, and let them know they are safe with you. Now it is time to reparent your inner child. Once your inner child is open to speaking freely, you can deepen the conversation in the new safe space you have created together.

Reparenting was introduced in the 1970s by Dr. Lucia Capacchione through art therapy. This technique focuses on showing your inner child they are loved, protected, and accepted in a way they lacked in their adolescent years. A large part of our personality stems from the power that our inner child holds over us into adulthood, in our thoughts, relationships, decisions, and how we approach situations and interpret them. Now is the time to reintroduce techniques to your inner child to minimize the negative loops that cause you anxiety and the mindset that is closing you off from acceptance of a productive and happy life.

Ways to Begin a Healing Dialogue With Your Inner Child

As with any new relationship, you may not know how to dive in and get a dialogue going. It often helps to put to paper what is bothering us about ourselves or someone else, because it helps release what we've been holding onto and are too afraid to say. The same can be done with your inner child. To begin, you will need to have two pieces of paper ready (envelopes optional), but don't worry about sending them anywhere, as they are only meant to release the pain and begin healing.

You will be writing one letter as your inner child to those who made them unworthy or ignored as a child and then a second from yourself to your inner child.

Letter From the Inner Child to the People/Person Who Caused Trauma

The letters you send from your inner child should have no boundaries so the inner child can say exactly what they need to. Address the people in your life who hurt you, abandoned you, or made you feel shame. Say anything you kept inside when you were young. Let all the pain out without holding back. Allow your inner child to say all they were too afraid to say when they had no voice.

There should be nothing unsaid and no worries about anyone else's feelings, because no one will ever read your letter. This is a healing process that will only help if you allow your inner child to direct their anger at those who hurt them most when they were too small to stand up for themselves. There is no need to explain your inner child's feelings; just say what you need for their tiny voice to finally be heard.

Letter to Your Inner Child

When you write to your inner child, you need to be careful with your words. Your words to this child will be absorbed completely and will redirect how they behave and interact with you. Give your inner child the compassion and validation they never received when they were young.

Begin by acknowledging the suffering your inner child endured. This will let them know that you see them, you hear them, and you will always be there for them. Adamantly deny them of any wrongdoing and help alleviate the guilt they might have been carrying all this time. They are not to blame for any of the pain they've been holding onto, and none of the unpleasantness they felt was because they were bad or inadequate. Let them know you are going to help protect them and help them move beyond their pain, but make sure they know they can always bring it up if need be.

Tell your inner child that they are brave for speaking to you now and strong for showing such vulnerability. Reinforce that you will always be present for them and will remain a steadfast guide of love in their life.

Speak Aloud to Your Inner Child

Some use a mirror to speak directly to themselves during this exercise, but you do not have to. You do need to ask your inner child questions out loud, speaking to your reflection or just to the air. Answer the questions truthfully and without restraint. If you feel emotional, comfort your reflection or yourself.

Use words you never heard when you were young, words that you wish had been said to you to soothe you or make you less afraid or feel more loved.

Write in a Journal or Diary as Your Inner Child or Adult

Dr. Lucia Cappachione, author of *The Power of Your Other Hand: A Course in Channeling the Inner Wisdom of the Right Brain*, suggests using your dominant hand to write as the adult and non-dominant hand for the inner child when journaling. This technique, according to Dr. Cappachione, engages the right brain, which is connected to emotional expression.

The dominant hand is that of the adult and should be used to write things to let the inner child know they are heard and are safe. The non-dominant hand should speak as the wounded inner child who is just discovering a way to speak for themselves. Your mind will distinguish the conversation between the two personalities using opposite hands that represent each half of you as they work together to become whole and learn about each other.

Artistic Expression

When you were a child, what made you really excited? What inspired you or made you feel that you could do anything? Whether through singing, dancing, drawing, or writing, these creative expressions help create a place of escape where you feel calm and safe.

Communicate in a way that makes you feel heard and in a space that allows you to become lost in the activity. Using artistic expression rather than words can be a powerful way to bring your emotions to the surface and allow them to be faced with honesty. The more in tune your inner child is with the activity, the more outpouring of creative energy and emotion can be released.

Make Time to Play With Your Inner Child

Your inner child needs to come out to play from time to time, and you need to be ready and willing to go on the adventure alongside them. When you feel a lighthearted or childish moment coming on, embrace it and the joy of freedom you once felt.

Watching shows, reading books, or revisiting places you loved as a child can help pull you back into a carefree world that was colorful and animated and limitless when you were younger. No activity is off limits as long as it's safe. Go play on the swings, go puddle jumping, or have a snowball fight. Reintroduce yourself to the unbridled joy of your inner child when they found their happy place.

Nurturing Your Inner Child as the Parent You Needed

Nurturing your inner child and showing them the compassion and love you wish you had as a child is essential for taking back your life. How can you parent yourself the way you wish you were parented or protected by the adult in your childhood? To answer this question, you need to ask yourself the following to determine what your wounded inner child needs:

- Is it a safe place?

- Is it acceptance?

- Do you need to be recognized for what makes you special?

- Do you need someone to stand up for you?

- Do you need emotional validation?

- Do you need to be heard?

- Do you need to feel that someone was proud of you?

Some ways to help yourself receive this inner validation include the following:

- **Have a safe place.** Everyone needs to feel safe, and routine is a positive way to promote that feeling. Safety can come in many forms, from how we make our home to the company we keep, but it can also come in the form of rituals that we perform each day to remind ourselves of the stability we have created. This ritual may include taking a walk through the same park each day or having a morning coffee while reading the paper. How we feel safe is personal, so find your safe space, ritual, or people, and visit at least once a day.

- **Be accepted.** You may not feel accepted because of mistakes you made in the past, but that needs to change. Everyone has done something they wish they could take back, whether it was done intentionally or not.

- **Learn from your mistakes and spin them into something that is more positive in the future.** If you do falter, simply ask yourself what you could do differently next time. Do not dwell on the misstep but on the positive steps you can take to create a different outcome in the future. This is known as a fixed mindset.

- **Envelope mistakes and use them for learning purposes.** Write down times you judge yourself and are self-critical, and then see how these outlooks can be shifted into a more positive form of acceptance. Things may not shift to the fixed mindset immediately, but with practice, you will accept yourself and all your beautiful mistakes.

- **Recognize what makes you unique.** Children are innately curious and seek out answers to the observations they make about the world around them, but sometimes they blurt out rather embarrassing statements about individuals who may appear different, such as

  - Why is that man yelling?

  - Why does that woman have only one leg?

  - Does that kid need to stay in that wheelchair forever?

  These are all valid questions, and they should be asked. Children tend to feel awkward that they don't belong to the restrictions we put on what they may ask of others or what others may ask of them. If your child has engine red hair and freckles, wore glasses from an early age, was born with one arm, or has some other unique trait, they need to feel comfortable about it.

  Just as a child deserves to feel special for their unique qualities, so do you. Write down a list of your unique traits, talents, features, etc., and then write something fascinating about it. If you have dyslexia, guess what? So do Henry Winkler, Anderson Cooper, and Albert Einstein!

  Embrace your uniqueness! You're already one of a kind, so anything extra just proves how amazing you are.

- **Validate your emotions.** Much distress in the inner child comes from adults not allowing them to display emotions. They are often perceived as having weakness or bad behavior and are told not to cry or say certain things when they are mad but just to forget about the experience and move on. This invalidates a child and makes a lasting impression on an inner child that moves forward through adulthood.

Don't push your feelings away when they come to you. If you're angry or disappointed, allow yourself to feel these emotions without judgment or reaction. Your feelings need to be acknowledged at the moment because you have a right to feel what comes naturally to you. Without telling yourself to stop feeling, soothe yourself as you would have wanted your parents to do when you were young. Tell yourself you understand these feelings are valid and you will sit as long as you need.

Don't allow shame to become any part of your reaction to what you're going through. When the adults around you said you were a failure, or a baby, or whiny, or not good enough, it was they who were wrong. Remember you were taught to feel shame and undeservedly so. You are not perfect and you do have flaws—as does everyone—so accept it and feel your feelings.

- **Be heard.** A child's voice is small, but it has as much to say as anyone else. Perhaps you felt no one listened to you when you were small, whether it was about what you wanted for dinner, where you wanted to go on vacation, or how you felt about moving away from your home or school.

  Sit your inner child down and apologize on behalf of the adults who never acknowledged what they had to say, and assure them you are listening now. Recount each time you didn't feel you had a voice and validate each experience so your inner child knows they are not silenced anymore. Ask your inner child how they felt, why they felt that way, and what they would have liked the adult in their life to do differently. Give that to them now.

- **Feel proud of you.** Many children spend what should be the happiest years of their lives struggling to find acceptance within their own space: their home. The family that should support them and love them expresses disappointment no matter how hard they try.

You were made to feel your accomplishments weren't enough and, in turn, you weren't enough. Perhaps you got a B- that you worked especially hard for but were asked why you didn't get an A? Or you came in second in a relay and your dad scoffed that you should have trained harder to be number one. No matter what you did, it wasn't enough, so you felt ashamed and that you would never live up to expectations.

Tell your inner child they were enough, their triumphs were in trying at all, and they should be proud of their achievements because you couldn't be more thrilled with their efforts.

Make a list of all the sports, teams, and adventures you were a part of during your childhood, and name your favorite thing about each one as well as something you were really good at. Tell yourself how proud you were back then and how nothing about that has changed.

Rewrite the Future With a Behavioral Experiment

Psychotherapists also suggest clients conduct behavioral experiments that test their beliefs. It is a powerful technique used in cognitive behavioral therapy that helps provide clarity to one's assumptions, rather than seeing things from only their perspective.

If you only believe one thing for sure, you may be ignorant of the truth, such as what actually happened, who did what, or how things transpired. Holding onto your beliefs unequivocally can mislead you.

For example, someone who believes they will be overweight because there is a family history of obesity and related illnesses may be encouraged to try a variety of ways to maintain a healthy weight, such as

o   exercising

- o eating healthy
- o getting plenty of rest

How the Experiment Works

Cognitive behavioral therapists, as mentioned previously, work with people to help them recognize their issues and the emotions, thoughts, and beliefs about these issues or problems. The therapist then helps the patient identify false thoughts and patterns that make the issue worse.

The next step is to help the person challenge their illogical and unproductive thoughts through the processes of questioning them and encouraging them to think of other ways to see the issue at hand.

Questions need to be asked by the therapist that helps the patient see deviations from their presuppositions. For example, a therapist might ask a client who feels they can't do anything to remember a time when they did something really well.

This simple form of questioning can help the patient realize they are not entirely accurate in their assumptions.

When someone believes deeply that they are a certain way or that something is entirely true, it can be challenging to change the thought patterns around these core beliefs, partly because we are more ready to see evidence that supports what we think instead of what proves us wrong.

If someone believes they have no skills and then gets rejected for a job they applied for, they may consider this proof that they are not good at anything. Alternatively, if they are invited out with a group of friends, they may consider this out of sympathy and not because they like their company.

Someone may begin to believe in their abilities when they accomplish something they never thought they could, such as completing a triathlon or getting a promotion. Likewise, if someone gets a positive response from someone they assumed would put them down, they may release the thoughts that everyone is untrustworthy.

Behavioral experiences can help build up self-esteem by gathering proof they are capable and may help them see the good in the world.

The Experiment

There are many ways to perform behavioral experiments. Some people may conduct a survey to gather proof of what others believe. Some may want to confront their fears head-on.

No matter which behavioral experiment the person is directing, the client and therapist work together on the exercise by

- recognizing the exact belief, process, or thought the experiment will focus on.
- brainstorming to come up with ideas for the analysis.
- predicting and formulating a method to document the outcome.
- forecasting challenges and brainstorming to generate solutions.
- orchestrating the experiment.
- reviewing and drawing conclusions on the experiment.
- discerning if additional experiments are required to follow up.

The client, along with their therapist, will propose the experiment, and then conduct it and monitor the results closely. Then they discuss the results and how they impact the client's beliefs.

The therapist may recommend further analysis or experiments to form a stricter assessment of the client's unhealthy beliefs.

Examples of Experiments

- Psychotherapists can help individuals formulate a behavioral experiment that can neutralize most skewed thoughts. Some examples of these behavioral experiments are below:

- A woman feels tired at bedtime so she stays on social media and watches videos until she falls asleep. Her behavioral experiment requires her to stop taking her phone or other electronics into her room at night and see if she feels more restful reading a book before bedtime instead.

- A man suffering from depression stays in his bed on days when he is particularly down. He spends the day on his phone or watching television and leaves his bedroom only to get food. The behavioral experiment requires him to get out of bed and go to work, spend the day with friends, or be productive.

- A woman feels her life is inadequate because she sees social media posts of her friends seemingly living exciting and perfect lives. She checks what her friends post every day. Her behavioral experiment requires her to stay off social media for an entire week to see if she feels less envious of the lives others lead.

- A man worries that people only like him because of what he can offer them. He is afraid to say "no" to anything people ask of him, even when he doesn't have the time. His behavioral experiment requires him to say "no" when someone asks him to do them a favor and see how they respond.

- A woman believes her friends only hang out with her because she likes to treat them to coffee, dinner, and other social outings. She doesn't say "no" because she is worried they won't hang out with her anymore. Her behavioral experiment requires her not to pay for the tab next time she is out with her friends and see how they react.

Building Emotional Intelligence

Emotional intelligence (EI) refers to the ability to use, perceive, manage, and understand your emotions. When you possess these abilities, you are more likely to benefit from academic achievement, solid decision-making, and personal and professional success. It can be argued that emotional intelligence is more likely to benefit your life than a high intelligence quotient (IQ).

What exactly is emotional intelligence? It is the capacity to perceive, interpret, control, demonstrate, and to use emotions when communicating in a constructive and effective way with others.

What Is Required for Emotional Intelligence?

How can we become emotionally intelligent? Psychologist Brandon Goleman, who made the concept popular in his book Emotional Intelligence, suggests five components of emotional intelligence. They are as follows (Goleman, 2005):

Self-awareness: The capability to acknowledge and understand one's emotions is a highly important skill when reaching emotional intelligence. Along with recognizing one's emotions is the ability to know the effect your moods, emotions, and actions have on others.

Monitoring your emotions is key to becoming self-aware, including observing your own emotional reactions and identifying each of them. Someone who is self-aware is able to recognize the connection between their feelings and how they behave. They also know their own limitations and their strengths and readily invite new experiences, learning from their exchanges with other people.

Dr. Goleman states that those who are self-aware are confident and are at ease with others, displaying social awareness and identifying social cues. Those who are self-aware are under no delusions as to how others perceive them.

Here are some ways to improve upon your own self-awareness:

- meditate
- write down your thoughts and interactions
- invite constructive feedback
- try new things
- set goals
- be aware of your emotions and thoughts behind them
- be mindful
- engage in positive self-talk
- look back on personal experiences
- allow your mindset to grow

Social skills: Interacting with others in social and work situations is vital to having healthy emotional intelligence. Strong social skills help build significant relationships and develop greater potential to understand ourselves and others.

Understanding your emotions and those of others is a part of social skills, but you also need to utilize this information when you interact with others to communicate appropriately.

In a work setting, for example, if you can connect with coworkers or your employees effectively, you will create a more successful work environment. Some important social skills include

- nonverbal communication skills
- verbal communication skills
- active listening
- persuasiveness
- leadership

If you can build a strong relationship with people you associate with in your work life and social life, you are more likely to build stronger bonds and be able to move forward with a relationship that creates efficiency. You can improve your social skills by

- asking open-ended questions
- being aware of others' social skills
- practicing comfortable eye contact
- using commonalities or ice breakers to begin conversations
- showing you are interested in what others say or do
- practicing active listening skills
- being aware of your body language
- working on your social skills

Self-regulation: It is important to be aware of our emotions and how they affect others; it is equally important to regulate our emotions and manage how we present them to others. By no means should you hold in your feelings and lock them deep inside, but it does refer to waiting for the opportune moment to express them. Self-regulation is an important tool for communicating your feelings appropriately.

When someone is able to self-regulate, they adapt better to challenging circumstances and change without issue. They also tend to be more considerate of how they might impact others and be willing to take control of their own actions and hold themselves accountable for how they behave.

You can become adept at self-regulation by practicing the following:

- being aware of your feelings and thoughts
- managing challenging emotions
- considering obstacles as opportunities
- working on communication skills
- having efficient communication skills
- improving distress tolerance
- accepting your feelings
- recognizing that you choose to respond the way you do
- applying cognitive reframing to disrupt emotional responses and thought patterns

Motivation: Intrinsic motivation offers a reward for our actions that are motivated by the satisfaction within. Those who have emotional intelligence are driven by the reward of inner satisfaction rather than external rewards such as money, fame, or recognition.

These people have a desire and drive to achieve their goals because of the rush they get or the feeling of the experience. They tend to be driven, take initiative, and set high standards for themselves when determining what they are able to achieve.

Ways to improve your motivation include

- acknowledging your results
- pushing yourself to stay interested
- aiming to achieve small, clear, and measurable goals
- not using extrinsic rewards
- setting attainable goals and building intrinsic motivation

Empathy: The ability to share feelings with and understand other people—empathy—is essential to emotional intelligence. Empathy is more than recognizing the emotions of others, however. It involves how you respond to people based on the information you have.

How do you respond to someone who is feeling anxious or worried? Someone with empathy would try to calm them down and let them know that everything will be okay.

Empathy equips you to better understand the dynamics that impact social relationships, particularly in the workplace. They help guide your exchanges with those you face every day. When someone is able to sense who holds the power in various dynamics, they can decipher various situations that depend on these power dynamics.

Build empathy by

- listening to others

- engaging in conversation with new people
- putting yourself in someone else's shoes
- doing community service or helping with a community event
- expressing and sharing your feelings
- practicing meditation

The Importance of Emotional Intelligence Skills

Having strong emotional intelligence skills can positively impact a person's life. Those who possess this skill tend to remain level-headed in difficult situations, handle uncomfortable situations well, and make others feel more comfortable.

Benefits of strong emotional skills include the following:

o   Leadership: Emotional intelligence creates a more constructive and persuasive leader.

o   Self-knowledge: When you are aware of your feelings, it allows you to understand yourself on a deeper level.

o   Self-control: When you are in control of your emotions, you are able to develop skills that allow you to control your reactions to those emotions.

o   Communication: Learn to understand others and how they are feeling. This will enable you to communicate with them more effectively.

o   Stress management: When you are able to control your emotions, you have more control during circumstances that are stressful or filled with conflict.

Emotional intelligence allows you to feel more empathy for those around you which allows you to better develop and maintain interpersonal relationships. Creating stronger bonds with people creates a support network in your life that is essential for mental and emotional wellness.

Activities to Build Emotional Intelligence

You know what it takes to foster emotional intelligence, so now we're going to look into activities that can help build emotional intelligence.

Actively Listen

Nonverbal communication can be just an important method of conveying our emotions as verbalizing them, therefore, we must watch for both positive and negative reactions to what we are conveying.

We have all experienced the feeling that someone is hearing words come out of our mouths but not actually understanding what we are saying. When you demonstrate that you are listening to what someone has to say, it will build a deeper connection, and respect, and lay the foundation for a meaningful relationship. To be a good active listener, ask questions, repeat key points, or nod on occasion to show you are paying attention to the meaning of their words.

Journal

Journaling is a good tool for keeping in touch with your emotions and releasing pent-up negativity while strengthening your emotional intelligence. Writing your experiences and the thoughts and emotions you feel because of them is a productive and effective way to sift through issues as you go through your days. Journaling helps you to solve problems, gain more clarity on situations, and manage stress.

Effectively Communicate

Not only is clear communication a critical skill for emotional intelligence. Knowing what and how to say something and when to present the information are all equally important. A team leader must be clear when communicating what they expect of the team and keep everyone up to speed on the goals. Be honest and concise in your communication, don't mince words, and provide an open mind for others to communicate their feelings to you.

Acknowledge the Feelings of Others

Being in tune with yourself and expressing your thoughts and feelings is important, but so is being aware of how others perceive the way you behave and how you communicate. You may be a direct person, but if you are blunt to a fault, you may be perceived by some as abrasive. If you are unsure of how others regard you, it's okay to ask; in fact, it will show them that you value their feelings.

Stay Positive

Maintaining a positive and calm disposition, even when things are hectic, will help those around you. Staying positive in difficult situations can be a lifeline to others that may be feeling stressed. We all indulge in negative feelings occasionally, but when we have a proactive approach, we have more power to turn a bad situation around and advocate for an adequate solution.

Activities you can do to maintain a positive state of mind include the following:

- listening to music that makes you happy
- practicing a form of art such as dancing, painting, or playing guitar
- doing deep breathing exercises in chaotic situations

Maintain an Open Mind

Emotionally intelligent individuals are more approachable because they consider situations from the perspective of others. These people are also open to trying new ideas and implementing strategies that are outside the box. Instead of dismissing a new concept immediately, consider what it might look like if you incorporate it into your own life or work.

Confirmation bias is one of the cognitive reasons for many to be closed-minded. This is the tendency to look for, interpret, support, and then recall data in ways that support or confirm your beliefs. A step to defeating this bias is to acknowledge it and then take a moment to digest new information and evaluate it based on research and facts, rather than agreeing because it supports your beliefs.

To have confidence in your intellect and in your choices is commendable, but resolution in only your own ideals can be a sign of closed-minded thinking. Being open-minded requires you to question others, as well as yourself. As new information is learned, ask yourself if the source of the information is trustworthy. Have you considered other possibilities? Do you know a lot about this topic? Are you biased to the outcome of your thinking on this matter?

Consider information and how you can approach it open-mindedly, rather than reacting immediately. This requires more self-control and takes more effort, but it will offer an insight into other people's thinking and help you gain perspective on different views.

Research has shown that being knowledgeable or expert on a topic can make people closed-minded. The brain is imperfect and is continually learning, while technology, nutrition, medicine, and most other concepts and things on Earth are ever-changing, so no one truly knows it all. Believing you know everything about a topic can lead to ignorance or overestimation of your knowledge because your limits are not being acknowledged. Take a moment to hear other points of view and additional information that you may not be aware of, allowing everyone to learn something new and communicate in a cohesive way.

Some ways to implement an open mind are below:

Empathize

Try to maintain an open mind when dealing with others. You may not consider something they are going through to be particularly difficult, but all emotions are subjective. Whether you feel the same way or not, try to see situations from the other person's perspective and acknowledge how it feels to be in their shoes.

Respond to Constructive Criticism With Self-Reflection

Have you ever heard the expression, "Step outside of yourself"? The ability to take constructive criticism is the ability to hear what others have to say about your performance, how you handle a situation, and what you can do to react or convey things differently. Whether it's how you respond to feedback on your performance at work or the reaction when a friend confides in you, it's worth hearing what someone has to say from their perspective. Listening to what someone else has to say will allow you to acknowledge your faults and take responsibility for your decision.

Building Emotional Intelligence

You have learned the activities that can help you build emotional intelligence. Now, it's up to you to follow through on these steps.

Empathize: What have you done to show your inner child or others empathy?

Identify: What negative thoughts, expressions, or emotions are holding you back? How are you going to keep them under control?

Evaluate: What actions, relationships, and behaviors need to be rectified? What will your first step be

Express: How do you feel and why? What are you going to do to resolve any negative feelings?

Learning from past

Now that you have met your inner child, heard what they had to say, and let them know you will protect them, you need to make sure you can fulfill that promise. How can you put the lessons you have learned to good use? How can you build a better life where their growth is encouraged?

Having a traumatic childhood can cause post-traumatic stress disorder (PTSD) and can make seemingly simple tasks or situations terrifying. To protect your inner child, you need to find a way to set those boundaries and stick to them for stability.

For example, when someone gives you constructive criticism on your cooking, focus on the positives they offer and not just the negatives. When you give constructive feedback, compliment one or two things you like about their story, cooking, or clothing before offering criticism. Hearing the positive makes hearing what you need to work on easier.

A Guide to Setting Boundaries

Setting boundaries is vital for people who suffer from post-traumatic stress disorder (PTSD), but it can be difficult to do. Many who live with PTSD also bear feelings of shame, guilt, and unworthiness, making it difficult for them to set boundaries to protect themselves. When others do not respect their boundaries, it can cause further stress.

We cannot expect everyone to know immediately what our boundaries are, since we do not wear them expressly on our person. It can be awkward and challenging to set boundaries and even more so to communicate them to others, but this is also an essential step toward promoting your mental health and well-being.

When you set boundaries, you are setting up an invisible shield meant to protect your emotional, physical, and mental health. We often set boundaries for

- o emotions
- o thoughts
- o personal space
- o time
- o possessions
- o sexuality
- o ethics
- o culture
- o religion

Everyone should set the five main boundaries below within their personal and professional lives:

Physical: This refers to your personal space and how comfortable you are with someone touching you or even being close to you. Someone in your life may be very comfortable sharing shows of affection in public, but you may find even hand-holding awkward. This also means you need to be respectful of others' preferences.

Intellectual: These boundaries are the beliefs, concerns, and thoughts that you have. When someone does not regard these beliefs, they are being disrespectful.

Sexual: This refers to what you feel is appropriate or what you are comfortable with in intimate situations. You are allowed to express yourself if you find a form of touch or expression uncomfortable.

Emotional: This refers to what you are comfortable sharing with others, whether it is your feelings or your past. You are in charge of determining how much or how soon you divulge.

Financial: This boundary is all about money and how comfortable you are sharing your finances. You may want to avoid going on vacation with someone who spends money freely when you are on a budget. You may want to speak about how much money you have to someone you know is on a tight budget.

Everyone should feel they deserve to set boundaries that others need to abide by. Boundaries help build healthy relationships because they set rules for negotiating professional or personal relationships. The challenge can be to know where to begin putting up those dividers between what you will accept and what you will not tolerate. Boundaries can also help nurture

- o independence
- o emotional strength
- o self-esteem

Setting boundaries may sound like you are setting up a wall around yourself and not letting anyone in, but the truth is that boundaries, such as the below, set a parameter to respect and acknowledge one another's feelings:

Improve self-esteem: When you set a boundary, you are protecting yourself from having relationships become precarious. The limits placed on ourselves and others help our relationships maintain a closeness while allowing you to put precedence on your own health, whether within your career, personal relationships, or your own self-care.

By establishing personal boundaries, you are demonstrating how you have become more responsible for your life. You are in control of how you will be treated by others and will react in a way that reinforces your boundaries. The more you demand respect and consideration from others, the more you will begin to see yourself as being worth it.

Preserve emotional energy: When you are unable to advocate for yourself, your self-esteem can be affected and you may begin to resent those around you. There is no rule that you need to set the same boundaries for everyone in your life. Navigate the settings of your boundaries depending on the situation or the people or person that you associate with.

If your mental wellness is suffering because you are bearing the emotional brunt of a friend's personal drama, you need to alleviate yourself of that negative energy. This doesn't mean that you are not able to help that same friend out when they need help moving homes.

Allow for flexibility: You may find that at the beginning of your healing journey or at various times in your life, you need to set stricter boundaries than at other times. Don't feel that once a limit is set, you are unable to loosen it. Being too strict on boundaries may cause you to become isolated, or it may cause you to abandon them altogether.

Allow room to grow and the opportunity to be vulnerable: Life is complicated, as are feelings at various stages and during certain events in our lives. Setting boundaries that you will release at the right time is revealing your vulnerability.

A display of vulnerability can be speaking about a difficult time in your life to your friends. Showing that you trust someone enough to open up about your feelings will show them that they can feel comfortable opening up to you, should the need arise.

There is a difference between sharing too much and being vulnerable. When we are vulnerable, we allow ourselves the opportunity to create a common bond with someone, but when you overshare, you risk dramatizing a situation or using it to manipulate the relationship to go in a certain direction.

Ways you may be sharing too much are below:

- You release your issues onto anyone who will listen.

- You are the only one speaking in the conversation.
- You air your drama or anger on social media.
- You expect people to be a part of your drama at a whim.
- You share too much information with a new associate or friend.

Setting boundaries on communication is important for yourself as well as others. When you share too much information, you may push someone out of their comfort zone and create unnecessary distance in your relationship rather than bring you closer together.

Setting and Maintaining Healthy Boundaries

Setting new boundaries does not mean you have to abandon your existing ones. You may need to revisit boundaries at a later date as circumstances change and you grow, but that is up to you to do on your terms in alignment with what makes you comfortable. Some simple ways to begin include:

Take time for self-reflection: Introducing boundaries isn't as simple as spewing off some nos and don'ts. It is important to understand and acknowledge why you are setting each boundary and how it will benefit you emotionally. Discover what makes you uncomfortable by diving into your own psychological needs. You don't need to set them all at once either, but gradually implement what works best for you and helps to protect the safety of your inner child.

Take small steps: Set your boundaries gradually rather than all at once. You may not realize what you need to limit until a situation occurs, so don't feel that you need to decide all at once. Setting a few limits at a time can be impactful and allow you to reflect on your decisions and determine if you are heading in the direction that works for you.

Set boundaries early in a relationship: Setting boundaries once you are already in a relationship can be challenging. Set boundaries at the beginning and there will be less chance of confusion, frustrations, or hurt feelings.

Be consistent: Once you loosen your boundaries, either because someone guilts you into it or because it's easier for you, you are opening the door to others demanding more of you. Keep things consistent and the line between what you will accept and not accept remains drawn.

Add boundaries to existing ones: In many situations, boundaries are already set, such as at a workplace, but this doesn't mean additional ones cannot be added to make you feel more comfortable. There may be a no dating policy between coworkers, but you can take this a step further and decline any invitations to outings that do not pertain to the workplace. Some people prefer to keep their work life completely separate from their personal life.

Communicate clearly and effectively: If someone is constantly ignoring your boundaries, you need to clarify them. This may be uncomfortable, but it doesn't need to be confrontational. If you have a sibling or friend who expects you to babysit regularly, there is nothing wrong with telling them you have plans but would babysit another time you are free.

Monitor social media posts: It is easy to be a keyboard warrior or express your problems on social media because it allows a sense of anonymity. It can also be tempting to chime in when others share their personal stories, but you may find this opens up the door for others to pry into your life and push your boundaries more than you are comfortable with. If you do not feel good about telling a stranger about your issues in person, it's likely not a good idea to post them on a social platform for all to see.

Advocate for yourself: When setting boundaries, be an advocate for what you deserve. If you think little of yourself, you are likely to be wary of demanding a certain level of respect or privacy, for example. Set a dialogue in your head saying you are good enough for the respect you demand from others. It is not greedy of you to ask others to respect your privacy or not ask about certain aspects of your life. Doing something that will make you feel good and get serotonin levels rising will help boost your confidence and expect the respect you give to others.

Recognize That Other People Have Boundaries

As crucial as your boundaries are to you, there needs to be mutual respect for the limits set by other people about what they believe is best for them, even if they don't advocate for yours.

Recognizing the boundaries of someone close to you may be easy, such as a spouse, sibling, or child. If your loved one doesn't post pictures of themselves online, chances are you shouldn't either.

If you are unsure of someone's boundaries, ask them questions like the following:

Do you mind if I post that photo of us?

What time can I call you?

Are you okay if I talk to you about…?

Boundaries are critical for your emotional well-being and that of your inner child. When you are protecting yourself, you are also protecting them. These lines look different to everyone. Just as you wouldn't be comfortable with someone pushing your limits, you should respect others.

Limits are a healthy way to ensure you are not put into an awkward situation and are surrounding yourself with positive and uplifting scenarios and people. Nothing is ironclad, but changing your boundaries too frequently can result in none.

Knowing When Boundaries Need to Be Set

Being able to separate your feelings from another person's is what is meant by keeping boundaries. People have their own memories, thoughts, and experiences that can be overshared and blurred with another person's own life. Implementing boundaries helps keep that space healthy and just for you.

It is fairly easy to determine when your physical limits are infringed upon, but psychological and emotional boundaries are more difficult to determine when a line is crossed. You are going to have to trust your own feelings and intuition when it comes to where the line is drawn for those boundaries.

Recovering From Abandonment Issues

Those who suffer from abandonment issues are afraid of being left behind or abandoned by those they love. People are usually not preoccupied with the thought of their friends and family leaving them, but someone who has experienced this in the past, particularly in childhood, is more susceptible to these types of concerns.

You know that many things can cause abandonment issues and what that looks like, but it's time to heal from your traumatic past and begin a better future alongside your newest friend: your inner child.

Examples of how someone with abandonment issues might act are below:

- They are clingy in a relationship.
- They are overly eager to please everyone.
- They have difficulty trusting anyone.

Some ways for you to acknowledge your abandonment issues while preventing them from controlling your outlook on your life and disposition include the following:

Express your emotions: Your inner child's voice needs to be heard now. Talk openly in therapy, to a friend, or even to those who hurt or abandoned you if they will listen.

When you express your emotions, they are easier to process and move past. Once you have voiced what you must, you can close the door on that part of your life and move forward.

Recognize irrational fears: The fear of losing those close to you is something you are allowing to come between you and healthy relationships. Recognizing that you are not going to lose your loved ones will help you to catch these irrational thoughts and stop them from spiraling into a stream of relentless contemplation.

Repair internalized shame: When a child does not receive adequate love growing up, they experience internalized shame, which represents feelings of self-hatred, self-loathing, and self-disgust. These are intense feelings and thoughts of there being something wrong within.

Internalized shame can present in various forms or negative self-talk, such as:

- feeling you can't do anything right
- hating yourself
- repeatedly apologizing
- feeling you are a burden
- feeling guilty
- self-harming (drinking excessively, reckless driving, cutting)
- being critical of how you look
- feeling self-hatred or disgust
- feeling unworthy of love
- consistently feeling of embarrassed for yourself
- thinking about death

These feelings, in addition to feelings of inadequacy, seep into your core and construct your identity, denying you the experience of exploring life fully. Healing the shame you feel requires you to work on your inner core and find yourself.

You need to reinvent yourself, so to speak, and realize that you are whole and loved. You are not the shell of a child the adults in your life made you believe you were. You need to remind yourself of all you have and reset confidence within your core.

Build a Better Support Network

For any recovery, whether emotional, mental, or physical, a good support system is essential. Having a strong support network includes friends and family, but the roots of ensuring your mental health are optimal. You need a network that allows you to cover all aspects of your recovery journey.

Some people may struggle to build a support network, especially if they are new to an area, have few family and friends, or are reserved in what they share.

Recovery is an intimate and personal journey of empowerment and discovery, and your hopes and goals differ from everyone else. Many factors will contribute to how you overcome your painful past and reacquaint yourself with the world as a newly healed individual, but you may not want to try it alone.

A support system, built with people you trust, is going to help you through the times that see you relapsing on your journey. Family, friends, members of your faith, neighbors, coworkers, and support groups may help in different ways to help you build a stronger sense of self.

A support network can promote a stronger sense of security and have a positive influence on your mental health overall. If you are battling your past or trying to move onward with a new outlook, it will not do you any good to dwell

Setting Boundaries Worksheet

Setting boundaries is top priority in your relationships to maintain a healthy balance of respect on both sides. Understanding which boundaries you have particular trouble with and working on more strictly reinforcing them is key to healthy relationships.

1. Which boundaries do you find most difficult to uphold?

2. Do you find it challenging to set boundaries with specific people? Who are they?

3. What do you find most angering or frustrating about this person or persons?

4. Why do you find it so challenging to set boundaries with them?

5. What can be the first boundary to set with them?

Self care for the inner Child

On this path to self-discovery, you need to remind your inner child that things are going to be okay, that there are brighter days ahead, full of laughter and a new beginning.

It is always okay—and necessary—to keep your inner child alive and to acknowledge what they have gone through to bring you to the place you are now. But with the recognition of the pain, you need to celebrate the light moments you experienced in your childhood as well.

Keeping your inner child close to you is a way to appreciate the steps you've taken to bring you into adulthood. You are both responsible for the person you are today, and without one, there would not be the other. It is the most important connection you can have with anyone.

Maintaining a happy relationship with your inner child is ongoing. Celebrating the fun moments in life are what will allow you to maintain a strong mindset moving forward. Below are some tips to maintain a healthy relationship with your younger self and create a healthier outlook on life:

- **Be proud of your accomplishments:** Once you have completed a task, let yourself know you've done a good job. Acknowledge when you have made a good effort, even if not everything turned out perfectly. Your inner child needs to hear that they have done well and that today was a good day. Positive reinforcement encourages people to do well and to try again in the face of adversity. If you were too afraid, let your inner child know that they were brave for trying and that you will work with them tomorrow to get it done.

- **Let yourself know you are loved by yourself:** Love is a universal need, especially self-love. It feels amazing to know that someone loves you, but there is no greater satisfaction than feeling love within yourself. Even if you don't feel you deserve love, say it over to yourself until you believe it. You will be more open to the love of others once you accept your own.

- **Appreciate yourself:** Once you learn to appreciate yourself and acknowledge the work you have done to heal your mental state, provide food for yourself and your family, and work at the job you do, you will be more open to accepting the appreciation of others. If you don't see the value in yourself, chances are, you won't expect others to appreciate you either.

- **Acknowledge your worth:** You are an important part of the lives of many for what you do and for the bravery you have shown in carrying on in the face of adversity. Remind yourself you are worth all the kindness that comes your way.

Daily Affirmations for Your Inner Child

You have done the work to let your inner child know they are safe, protected, loved, whole, and wanted, and you have let them know you will not abandon or neglect them. You will need to continue to let them know that they are going to be seen and heard by you. These daily affirmations can help:

- "The pain of my childhood was real."

- "My feelings are valid."

- "I am worthy of love."

- "My younger self was not at fault."

- "Reparenting myself is helpful."

- "I deserve love."

- "It's okay to show emotions."

- "I am safe."

- "The voice of my inner child is valid."

- "I deserve respect."

- "I am worthy of my love and the love of others."

- "My self-worth is strong."

- "Expressing joy is the greatest gift to my inner child."

- "My inner child is free to laugh."

- "I love my inner child."

- "I am proud of who I was and who I am."

- "My inner child is happy."

- "I will no longer carry shame."

- "Today I will embrace only positive actions."

- "I trust myself."

- "I love who I have become."

- "I am whole.

- "The past should not be dwelled upon."

- "I will live each day in the present."

- "I am unstoppable."

Teachings From Your Inner Child

Healing your inner child is going to help you move forward with a greater sense of who you are and who your younger self should have been. Through reparenting your wounded inner child, you will hopefully come to repair some of the habits you have attained due to feeling inadequate and neglected.

Below are some ways that suggests you have healed your inner child wounds:

- You no longer feel inadequate; you know you are enough.

- Pleasing people all the time isn't possible or necessary.

- You once felt you needed conflict to feel alive, but you now know that harmony is a more productive and validating trait.

- Once a hoarder afraid of letting go of the past, you now know possessions do not replace emotions.

- Before, you struggled to keep relationships that were failing, but you now acknowledge that it's better to let some things go.

- You may still feel anxiety with new situations or people; however, you now acknowledge those feelings and go into a new situation with a positive attitude.

- You no longer feel guilt for setting boundaries; you now know that you deserve to protect yourself.

- No longer an overachiever, you now do what you can and make attainable and clear goals for yourself to complete in steps.

- Once a perfectionist, you know mistakes are to be learned from and incorporated into our life experiences.

- You had difficulty beginning and completing tasks, but now you set goals to complete them each day and follow through.

- Once, you were self-critical, but you now accept your flaws and move onward to be a better person.

- You used to avoid conflict, but you now stand up for yourself in a calm manner and don't back down.

- You had a fear of abandonment, but you have recognized this is an irrational fear and know that you are loved.

- Before, you were ashamed to express your feelings. You now know your feelings are valid and you should embrace them in appropriate settings and acknowledge them without pushing them down inside.

- You no longer body shame; you acknowledge that what makes you unique is beautiful.

- You distrusted everyone, but you now know not everyone is going to let you down.

Your inner child was compelling in shaping your emotions, beliefs, fears, emotions, and general conditioned thinking into your adult years. We know no one can go back and rewrite their childhood, but you can move forward with a new respect for the bravery and strength of your inner child and honor them by rising above the wounds that you suffered and making you and your younger self whole.

Repairing your mental health and maintaining it will allow you to have more positive experiences with your attachment to others and within yourself. You need to feel heard and know that someone understands you so that you find a more positive way to evaluate the history and progression of your life story. Nurturing your inner child and finding a positive outlook on your own life and how to negotiate relationships will help you move beyond the struggle you once felt.

Using calming techniques, confronting the way you see others, recognizing daily triggers, reclaiming your past, journaling, and other tools you have learned will allow you to compartmentalize your life into the two parts you now know: wounded inner child and strong adult. Your goal should be to acknowledge your inner child with compassion and move onward with the strength you have wielded throughout your life.

Acknowledge the sacrifices your inner child has made in exchange for simply getting by. They have taken responsibility for things they should not have, withheld feelings they should have been encouraged to share, and imagined trust rather than experiencing it. Now is the time to thank your inner child for their sacrifices, let them know you will always be there for them, and walk toward a more positive and well-deserved future for your adult self.

'Create a haven of safety within yourself, and watch as the world responds in kind.'

Marianne Williamson

———

CHAPTER SIX

Creating Safety and Stability

C hildhood trauma casts deep shadows, impacting every aspect of our lives. When trauma strikes during our formative years, it shatters our sense of safety and stability, leaving behind anxiety, fear, and relational challenges.

During your healing journey, we'll take on the essential task of creating safety and stability, laying the groundwork for healing and growth. Additionally, we'll delve into the intricacies of trauma, unraveling its effects on the nervous system and empowering you to identify triggers.

We'll forge a foundation of strength and resilience, charting a course toward personal transformation and renewed well-being. Step forward with confidence, knowing that you're not alone. This is your time to heal and thrive.

Understanding the Effects of Trauma on the Nervous System

Trauma experienced in childhood can leave profound effects on both your mental and physical health. However, the brain's capacity for neuroplasticity can facilitate the healing process.

Neuroplasticity describes our brain's ability to transform and adjust in response to external stimuli continuously. This phenomenon enables us to learn and adapt to new environments and experiences. Nonetheless, specific brain changes may lead to persistent physical and mental health complications in highly stressful circumstances such as traumatic events.

How Childhood Trauma Changes Our Brains

Throughout childhood, the brain exhibits high levels of plasticity, meaning that connections between different brain regions can shift in strength based on your childhood experiences and evolving understanding of the world. Unfortunately, many traumatic experiences during childhood are categorized as adverse childhood experiences (ACEs). These can include violence, neglect, abuse, and substantial disruptions that occur before turning 18.

According to Aebi et al. (2016), the experience of one or more ACEs can result in long-term impacts on a person's mental and physical health, which may increase the likelihood of developing

- depression

- anxiety

- antisocial behavior

- suicidal behavior

- impulse control issues

- attention deficit hyperactivity disorder (ADHD)

- post-traumatic stress disorder (PTSD)

- substance use disorder (SUD)

Childhood Trauma and Nervous System Sensitization

The amygdala, a small almond-shaped region in the brain, plays a crucial role in regulating emotions. For example, when it perceives a threat, it triggers a hypothalamus response, activating the sympathetic nervous system's "fight, flight, freeze, or fawn" response.

If you've experienced trauma as a child, you may have a more sensitive amygdala, causing you to perceive threats more readily. This hypersensitivity can make you more susceptible to experiencing depression, anxiety, and stress in adulthood.

Many people often feel embarrassed or ashamed by their heightened vigilance and sensitivity to mental disorders. This is enhanced by others often perceiving them as dramatic or a grandstander.

Regardless of other people's opinions, you're not alone in this. Hypersensitivity is quite common among those who have experienced childhood trauma. My own childhood forced me to suppress emotional expression, as I had to perpetually put on a brave face for my younger siblings and parents. As a result, my nervous system was sensitized, leaving me prone to heightened anxiety and hypervigilance. Little things, like my daughters approaching me from behind, will cause me to let out a yelp! These moments of exaggerated startle responses serve as a reminder that our experiences shape us in profound ways.

Childhood Trauma and Increased Inflammation

The sympathetic nervous system activation triggers our fight-or-flight response and our inflammation and immune system response. While these responses prepare the body for physical injury repair, they can also occur in response to psychological threats.

If you've experienced ACEs, you may have a higher risk of developing inflammation later in life. Additionally, your body may struggle to promote relaxation and prevent chronic inflammation. One study observing 1,000 individuals from birth to 32 years of age found a link between increased inflammation and childhood maltreatment (Danese & van Harmelen, 2017). When trauma causes inflammation, it can affect how neurotransmitters work in the brain and can impact brain development if it happens at a young age.

Healing Through Neuroplasticity

Neuroplasticity was once believed to be limited to early childhood, but modern brain imaging has shown that neuroplasticity is a lifelong quality. Hence, irrespective of your age, it is entirely within your capability to restructure your nervous system and rewire your brain, even in the face of childhood trauma, by cultivating fresh, nurturing, and affirmative experiences. Consider this process akin to forming new habits. By consistently engaging in the behaviors and immersing yourself in the experiences that align with your desired state, you can tap into the remarkable potential of neuroplasticity to your benefit. Through the intentional repetition of these constructive patterns, you have the ability to reshape your neural pathways, forge new connections, and foster profound healing and growth.

Identifying Triggers and Creating a Safe Environment

To successfully utilize neuroplasticity to create new positive experiences and develop new habits, it's essential to identify triggers that may cause trauma responses. Triggers can be anything from a sound or smell to a particular location or person. Identifying triggers can help you avoid them or prepare yourself to manage your response if you can't prevent them.

In addition to identifying triggers, creating a safe environment is crucial. A safe environment means creating physical and emotional spaces where you feel secure and comfortable.

Childhood Trauma Triggers

Although most people who experience traumatic events during childhood don't suffer long-term effects, many continue to be affected consciously or subconsciously throughout their lives. You may appear fine most of the time if you have a traumatic past, but certain circumstances can trigger your trauma-related symptoms to escalate dramatically. These symptoms are typically caused by exposure to trauma triggers, which are involuntary reminders of past trauma. Childhood trauma triggers include emotions, situations, smells, sights, and sounds.

Emotions

A specific emotion can be linked to the traumatic experience you had as a child, and particular situations in adulthood can trigger that emotion. For instance, encountering a problem that may seem manageable but makes you feel helpless can remind you of cases in which you were genuinely vulnerable as a child, leading to you becoming overwhelmed.

In addition to this, other examples of emotional triggers may include

- crying or experiencing sadness

- feeling abandoned

- being ignored

Situations

Sometimes, you might come across situations that bring back memories of a traumatic experience you had as a child. Some common circumstances that can trigger emotions include

- experiencing unwanted physical touch

- interacting with an authority figure

- feeling that your boundaries have been violated

- coming across someone with perceived narcissistic tendencies

- experiencing rejection

- driving a car

Sounds

Certain sounds have the potential to trigger unwanted responses that make our bodies feel unsafe, even when we are in a secure environment. For example, I grew up in a house where my parents would resort to shouting at the slightest inconvenience. Now, whenever someone raises their voice, even if it's due to happiness or excitement, it triggers negative memories of my parents. Some other common examples of sounds that can act as triggers include

- a car horn

- the sound of a door slamming

- a baby crying

- a specific musical instrument

Smells

Our senses are directly linked to our brains and constantly transmit messages as we interact with our environments. A particular scent can quickly bring up mental images and associated feelings. For instance, the smell of freshly cut grass might evoke memories of playing outside during the summer as a child.

Our brain immediately tries to identify the scent when we smell something. However, while it tries to identify the scent, it can also trigger memories of when we've previously encountered that same smell.

Some of the triggers that can result from smells include

- alcoholic drinks

- specific foods or non-alcoholic drinks

- fragrances or colognes

- gasoline

Sights

Witnessing a particular object, location, or individual can serve as a trigger, causing an unwarranted reaction. Suppose you experienced a traumatic event at a beach. In that case, being near a beach or viewing images of beaches may trigger negative emotions. These triggers could cause you to experience flashbacks or other trauma-related symptoms, even if you aren't in danger. Other examples of triggers can include seeing

- someone who resembles an abuser or attacker

- an object that was present during a traumatic event

- a particular color or pattern

- a specific hairstyle or physical feature of someone involved in the trauma

How to Identify Triggers

It's common for triggers to feel unpredictable, and they can sometimes be subtle and surprising. However, recognizing a trigger is the first step towards learning how to manage it.

One effective way to identify triggers is by starting a journal and recording your thoughts, emotions, and environment during flashbacks or panic attacks. You can ask yourself questions such as:

- What did you smell?

- What did you see?

- What did you hear?

- How were you feeling at the time?

You can identify your triggers by looking for patterns and similarities in your journal entries.

In a study conducted by Bryant et al. (2013), 46 trauma survivors were asked to maintain a daily journal to identify unwanted traumatic memories or potential intrusions. During the seven days, the participants reported a total of 294 intrusions. Surprisingly, the researchers found that the triggers leading up to these intrusive memories were often unknown to the participants.

The study's results highlight the importance of identifying triggers in managing trauma symptoms. When trauma survivors are unaware of their triggers, it can be challenging to anticipate and manage intrusive memories and associated emotional responses. However, by using tools like daily journals to identify and track their triggers, survivors can develop a greater awareness of their emotional responses and take steps to manage them. These steps may involve avoiding trigger situations or developing coping strategies to address the emotional response when a trigger is encountered. Identifying triggers is an essential step in healing from trauma and regaining control over one's emotional and mental well-being.

Creating a Safe Environment

Creating a safe environment for oneself after experiencing childhood trauma can be a complex and ongoing process, but it's absolutely crucial for healing, growth, and living a fulfilling life. It requires a combination of self-reflection, self-care, boundary-setting, and seeking support from others.

While each person's journey toward creating a safe space will be unique and personal, some general steps can be helpful to consider and implement in the process. By taking these steps, individuals can gradually feel more grounded, empowered, and safe in their everyday lives. Here are some steps that can help:

- Practice self-care: Taking care of yourself physically and mentally is essential. This encompasses prioritizing adequate sleep, nourishing your body with wholesome food, and immersing yourself in activities that bring you genuine joy and a sense of deep relaxation.

- Focus on mindfulness: Mindfulness practices such as meditation, deep breathing, and yoga can help you stay present in the moment and manage anxiety and stress.

- Surround yourself with supportive people: Seek out friends and family who are understanding and supportive. Joining a support group can also be helpful.

- Establish healthy boundaries: Set clear boundaries with others and communicate them effectively. This can include saying "no" to activities or situations that make you feel uncomfortable.

- Seek professional help: Working with a therapist or counselor who specializes in trauma can help you identify triggers and develop coping strategies.

It's crucial to remember that recovery is a gradual process that requires time. Throughout this journey, being kind and compassionate to yourself is vital. Recognize that small victories and steps are significant and should be celebrated. Any effort towards healing and growth is valuable and deserving of recognition.

Guided Relaxation and Grounding Exercises

This part of the book will explore techniques to help you relax, let go of tension, and find a sense of inner calm. These exercises will enhance your presence in the moment and your connection with your body. They are particularly beneficial for individuals who have experienced childhood trauma. So, whether you want to reduce stress and anxiety or deepen your self-awareness, these exercises can be a valuable tool in your healing journey.

To make the most of these exercises, I've created recordings of them for you to listen to. Accessing them requires you to open the camera on your smartphone or tablet and point it at the QR code. Your device will recognize the code and show a notification or a link. When you tap on the notification or follow the link, it will take you to Dropbox, where you can listen to or download the recordings. It's an easy way to access the exercises using your device and enjoy the benefits of relaxation and grounding.

Scan Me

Exercise 1: Body Scan Relaxation

This exercise combines deep breathing and a body scan to help you relax and release tension. By focusing on your breath and scanning your body for areas of tension, you can bring awareness to your physical sensations and release stress.

1. Find a peaceful and cozy area to unwind and avoid interruptions. Create a serene environment by dimming the lights or playing soft, soothing music if desired. Find a comfortable position that makes you feel relaxed and supported, whether sitting or lying down.

2. Close your eyes and take a moment to center yourself. Then, slow down your breath and concentrate on it. Next, inhale deeply through your nose and notice your stomach expanding as your lungs fill with air. Next, exhale slowly through your mouth, releasing tension or stress with each breath. Continue this deep breathing pattern a few more times, gradually letting go of any thoughts or distractions.

3. Take a moment to focus on your body. Start by directing your attention to the top of your head, then proceed systematically through each part of your body, making sure to give each area the attention it needs. First, notice any areas of tension, discomfort, or tightness that you may be holding. Then, with each breath, imagine sending a wave of relaxation to those areas, allowing them to soften and release any tension they may be having.

4. As you continue to breathe deeply and rhythmically, bring your attention to the sensation of your breath flowing in and out of your body. Notice how the air feels cooler as you inhale and warmer as you exhale. Pay attention to your chest or abdomen rising and falling with each breath. Concentrating on the present and disregarding any bothersome thoughts or concerns is essential.

5. Expand your awareness to your senses. What sounds are present in your surroundings? Is there a gentle hum, birds chirping, or the distant flow of water? Take a moment to fully listen to these

sounds, allowing them to wash over you and bring a sense of calm. Notice any pleasant aromas that may be present in the air, whether it's the scent of nature, a calming essential oil, or anything else that brings you comfort. Feel the sensation of the surface beneath you, whether a soft cushion, a supportive mattress, or the earth beneath your feet. Become aware of the textures, temperatures, and sensations on your skin.

6. Now, let your imagination take you on a journey. Visualize yourself in a peaceful natural setting of your choice. It could be a serene beach, a lush forest, a tranquil meadow, or any place that brings you a sense of tranquility. Take a moment to explore this setting in your mind's eye. Notice the colors, the textures, and the beauty of the surroundings. Feel the gentle breeze against your skin, the sun's warmth, or the grass beneath your feet. Immerse yourself in the experience and engage all of your senses.

7. As you bask in the serenity of this imagined place, allow yourself to experience a deep sense of relaxation and peace. Feel the stress and tension melting away, leaving you with a profound sense of calmness and tranquility. Stay in this state as long as you feel comfortable, savoring its peace and rejuvenation.

8. When you're ready, slowly bring your awareness back to the present moment. Wiggle your fingers and toes, gently stretch your body, and take a few deep breaths to awaken your senses. Carry this sense of relaxation and tranquility with you as you continue your day, knowing you can return to this practice whenever you need a moment of respite and rejuvenation.

Exercise 2: Mindful Breathing Meditation

This exercise aims to help you practice mindfulness using the square breathing technique. This technique involves breathing in for a specific count, holding your breath for the exact count, breathing out for that count again, and then holding your breath once more for the same count.

This exercise can help you feel calm, centered, and more aware of your breathing.

1. Begin this exercise by finding a quiet place to sit or lie down. Make sure you're comfortable by taking a moment to settle in and adjust your body. Place a blanket or pillow under your head or knees for extra support if needed.

2. To begin, get comfortable with your eyes open or closed. Next, take a deep breath through your nose and exhale slowly through your mouth. Let your breathing happen naturally, and avoid trying to manipulate it.

3. Now, as you inhale, count silently to four. Imagine breathing in peace and calmness, filling your body with relaxation and tranquility. Then, as you hold your breath for a count of four, feel the tension in your body starting to release and fade away.

4. Next, slowly exhale for six counts. Imagine releasing all the stress and tension from your body, letting go of any worries or concerns. Then, as you hold your breath again for a count of four, feel your body becoming lighter and more at ease.

5. Repeat this pattern for a few more cycles, allowing yourself to become fully absorbed in the rhythm of your breath. If you'd like, you can place your hand on your stomach to better sense your breathing pattern.

6. As you inhale and exhale, release any thoughts or distractions that may arise. If your mind wanders, guide your attention back to your breath. Relax and allow yourself to sink deeper into relaxation and inner peace.

7. To achieve a state of calm and peacefulness, try following this breathing pattern for a few minutes or as long as you'd like. To conclude the exercise, take a few deep breaths and gradually open your eyes as though they were closed. Finally, take a moment to recognize and assess your current emotional state. You may feel more at ease, grounded, or concentrated.

It's essential to take your time and adjust the count to a number that feels comfortable for you. The aim is to establish a pattern that makes you feel calm and centered. This exercise can be done anytime and anywhere if you need to relax and concentrate for a few minutes.

Exercise 3: Reorienting to the Present Moment

This exercise is designed to help you reorient yourself to the present moment by focusing on your senses. By engaging with your intentions and surroundings, you can ground yourself in the present and reduce feelings of anxiety or dissociation.

1. To begin, locate a calm and cozy spot to sit or lie down. Next, shut your eyes and take deep breaths, enabling you to unwind and release any bodily stress.

2. Now, bring your attention to your senses. First, notice the feeling of your body against the surface you're sitting or lying on. Next, tune in to the sounds around you—listen to the sounds that are far away, then the closer ones, then the ones that are nearest to you. Finally, take a few deep breaths and smell the scents around you.

3. Slowly start to move your body. Gently wiggle your toes and fingers, roll your shoulders, and stretch your arms and legs. If you're lying down, it's advisable to turn to one side slowly, then the other, and finally sit up slowly. Be mindful of your bodily sensations as you move, and stay aware of your surroundings.

4. Take a moment to observe your surroundings and identify the objects in the room. Take your time and reflect on each item. Then, if you're outside, name the things you see around you, such as trees, buildings, or clouds in the sky.

5. To feel more centered, take a few deep breaths and focus on your body. Notice how you're feeling and any changes in your body sensations. When you're ready, slowly open your eyes.

6. If you feel overwhelmed or disoriented, performing reorientation exercises can help you feel more grounded and present. Paying attention to your senses and surroundings can help your mind and body connect with the here and now and reduce feelings of anxiety or disconnection.

Exercise 4: Texture Exploration Exercise

This exercise aims to enhance your awareness and connection with the physical world using the sense of touch. By engaging your sense of touch, you can become more grounded and centered in the present moment and feel less overwhelmed by thoughts and emotions. This simple exercise can be done anywhere, at any time, whenever you need to feel more present and calm. You only require a small handheld object, like a coin or a stone, to start.

1. First, ensure you're in a comfortable position, sitting or standing. Take a few moments to release any tension in your body. Take a deep breath by inhaling through your nose and exhaling through your mouth. As you breathe, let go of any stress or anxiety you may be feeling.

2. Shift your attention to your sense of touch. Take a moment to concentrate on the sensation of your feet being securely placed on the ground, or the feeling of your body being upheld by the surface underneath you. Be mindful of how your clothing feels against your skin, the temperature of the surrounding air, and any other tactile sensations you may be experiencing.

3. Locate an object nearby that you can hold in your hand. It could be a stress ball, a smooth stone, or any interesting texture item. Take a moment to select an object that catches your interest.

4. Once you have the object in your hand, bring your full attention to it. Notice its weight and how it feels in your hand. Explore its texture, whether it's smooth, rough, or has any distinct features. Pay attention to any temperature sensations it may evoke.

5. Close your eyes and continue to engage your sense of touch. Experiment with different movements, such as rolling the object between your fingers, squeezing it gently, or rubbing it with your fingertips. Observe any sensations that arise and focus on the connection between your hand and the object.

6. As you continue exploring the object with your sense of touch, maintain a slow and steady breathing rhythm. Breathe deeply through your nose and slowly release the air through your mouth. Use the breath as an anchor, keeping you present and centered in the experience.

7. When you feel ready, slowly release the object from your hand and bring your awareness back to your surroundings. Take a moment to notice how your body physically feels when you concentrate on your sense of touch. Pay attention to changes in your relaxation, groundedness, or overall well-being.

8. If you find your mind wandering or anxious during your day, remember this exercise and the power of touch to bring yourself back to the present moment. Please take a few moments to repeat the exercise, focusing on the touch sensation and allowing it to anchor you in the here and now.

'Our core wounds are the tender places where we have been touched by life's challenges; embracing them leads to profound growth.'

Jack Kornfield

———

CHAPTER SEVEN

Identifying and Understanding Core Wounds

I n the previous chapter, we've learnt that experiencing trauma during childhood can profoundly affect a person's life in significant and enduring ways. Similarly, experiencing emotional trauma can cause long-lasting effects on a person's thoughts, feelings, and actions. These wounds, known as core wounds, can be challenging to identify and heal.

In fact, during the initial sessions with many of my patients, a significant focus is placed on identifying their core wounds. However, it's not uncommon for us to discover new wounds or gain a deeper understanding of existing ones much later in our journey together.

It takes a lot of courage and self-reflection to confront the pain and vulnerability of exploring these wounds. However, with patience, self-compassion, and the right tools, you can heal from the effects of your trauma and lead a fulfilling life.

How to Identify and Understand Your Core Wounds

Identifying and understanding your core wounds is essential in the healing process. By becoming aware of your past traumas and their impact on your present thoughts and behaviors, you can break free from their adverse effects and reclaim your power. You can identify and understand your core wounds in several ways, including through self-reflection, journaling, mindfulness practices, feedback from trusted others, and therapy.

Self-Reflection

Reflecting on your past experiences and relationships can be beneficial. First, look for patterns in your behavior and emotions. For example, identify moments when you felt hurt, rejected, or abandoned. Then, consider how those experiences have influenced your beliefs about yourself and your relationships.

I've found great success in taking a few minutes to explore the root cause of any negative emotions I feel, and I can typically trace them all the way back to my childhood. This practice has given me a better understanding of why events that others don't perceive as a big deal affect me so deeply.

Journaling

Jotting down your thoughts and emotions is an effective way to reveal hidden beliefs and recurring thought patterns. Write about your experiences, thoughts, and feelings related to relationships and identify recurring themes.

Mindfulness Practices

Engaging in mindfulness practices such as yoga and meditation can enhance your self-awareness and ability to observe your thoughts and emotions without judgment. Additionally, by being more present in the moment, you may better identify and understand your core wounds.

Feedback From Trusted Others

Consider asking your trusted friends or family members if they have noticed any recurring behavior patterns or have any insights about your core wounds. Getting an opinion from someone outside ourselves can give us valuable insight.

Therapy

Engaging in therapy can aid in delving into and comprehending your underlying traumas. Moreover, a therapist can assist in recognizing recurring thought and behavior patterns and offer encouragement while navigating through any emotional distress.

Examining the Negative Beliefs Associated With Core Wounds

Negative beliefs associated with core wounds can vary from person to person, as each individual's experiences and wounds are unique. However, the most common negative beliefs I've heard throughout my career include:

- "I am unlovable": Feeling unworthy of love and affection, believing that you're fundamentally flawed or undeserving of love and care.

- "I am not enough": Feeling a deep sense of insufficiency or lack, believing that you're not good enough, smart enough, attractive enough, or deserving of happiness.

- "I am powerless": Feeling helpless or powerless in various aspects of life, believing that you have no control or influence over their circumstances.

- "I am a failure": Holding a belief of being a failure or experiencing constant disappointment, believing that you're incapable of achieving your goals or living up to expectations.

- "I am unworthy of success": Feeling undeserving of achievement, believing that you're destined to fail or that success is reserved for others.

- "I am a burden": Feeling like a burden to others, believing that your needs and presence inconvenience or weigh down those around you.

- "I am unimportant": Feeling insignificant or unimportant, believing that one's opinions, feelings, and presence don't matter or hold value.

- "I am destined to be alone": Believing that meaningful connections and relationships are unattainable or that you're destined to be isolated and lonely.

- "I am always rejected": Expecting rejection or abandonment in relationships, believing that one is inherently unlovable or that others will inevitably reject them.

- "I am damaged beyond repair": Holding the belief that one's wounds and past experiences are irreparable, feeling permanently damaged or broken.

These negative beliefs can significantly impact self-esteem, relationships, and overall well-being. Therefore, identifying and challenging these beliefs to heal and create a more positive and empowering self-narrative is essential. One way to do that is through cognitive restructuring.

Cognitive Restructuring Techniques for Challenging Negative Beliefs

Cognitive restructuring is a valuable aspect of therapy that includes a range of techniques designed to help you identify and transform negative thinking patterns that are harmful and counterproductive. It plays a crucial role in disrupting and redirecting these patterns, aiming to promote healthier thoughts and behaviors. This widely-used form of cognitive-behavioral therapy has been extensively studied and demonstrated effectiveness in addressing various mental health challenges, such as anxiety and depression. By deconstructing unhelpful thoughts and reconstructing them in a more balanced and realistic manner, cognitive restructuring empowers you to cultivate a healthier mindset.

Within cognitive restructuring, the focus is on addressing cognitive distortions that many people experience. These distortions create false and unhealthy perceptions of reality, contributing to self-defeating behaviors, relationship challenges, anxiety, and depression. Common cognitive distortions include personalizing, overgeneralizing, catastrophizing, and black-and-white thinking. By engaging in cognitive restructuring, you can become more aware of these maladaptive thoughts as they arise and practice reframing them in more accurate and helpful ways. By shifting our perspective on events or circumstances, we can alter our emotional responses and subsequent behaviors, ultimately leading to positive change.

Cognitive Restructuring and Core Wounds

Cognitive restructuring plays a crucial role in the healing process of core wounds stemming from childhood trauma. By addressing and challenging the negative beliefs, distorted thinking patterns, and self-limiting narratives that arise from the trauma, cognitive restructuring promotes healing, resilience, and growth. Through this therapeutic approach, you can recognize that your traumatic experiences don't define your worth or determine your future.

In the process of cognitive restructuring, you're guided to confront and alter your negative fundamental beliefs about yourself, others, and the world around you. By carefully reviewing the evidence and considering alternative perspectives, you gradually shift your thinking towards more positive and empowering narratives. This transformative journey encourages the development of self-compassion, self-acceptance, and a sense of agency over your own life. With cognitive restructuring, individuals can reclaim their personal power and create a new narrative that aligns with their inherent worth and potential for a brighter future.

Cognitive Restructuring Techniques

Cognitive restructuring is typically conducted with a trained therapist's guidance. However, it's worth noting that cognitive restructuring can also be practiced independently.

In the following sections, we'll explore critical techniques that can aid in cognitive restructuring, including generating alternatives, performing a cost-benefit analysis, gathering evidence, Socratic questioning, self-monitoring, thought records, and decatastrophizing. These techniques offer practical tools for reshaping negative thinking patterns and promoting more positive and adaptive thoughts.

Generating Alternatives

Cognitive restructuring is a powerful technique that empowers you to reframe your thoughts and find new perspectives. By challenging negative or distorted thinking patterns, you can generate alternative explanations that are rational and positive.

For example, imagine you receive negative feedback on a project at work. Instead of immediately feeling defeated and thinking you're a failure, you could consider the feedback an opportunity for growth and improvement.

Similarly, let's say you experience a minor disagreement with your friend. Instead of jumping to conclusions and assuming they no longer value your friendship, consider alternative explanations. Maybe they had a busy day and were preoccupied or didn't fully understand your perspective. By taking different possibilities into consideration, it opens the door to healthier communication and understanding.

Generating alternatives can also involve challenging self-critical thoughts and replacing them with self-compassion and self-acceptance. For instance, if you make a mistake at work, instead of criticizing yourself, remind yourself that making mistakes is a natural part of learning and growth. Embrace a more compassionate perspective that allows for self-forgiveness and the opportunity to learn from the experience. By actively engaging in this technique, you can transform your thought patterns and cultivate a more positive and resilient mindset.

Performing a Cost-Benefit Analysis

Performing a cost-benefit analysis involves examining the advantages and disadvantages of maintaining a specific cognitive distortion. For example, reflect on the following questions:

- What do you gain from labeling yourself negatively?

- How does this thought pattern impact you emotionally and practically?

- What are the long-term consequences of holding onto this thought pattern?

- How does it influence the people around you?

- In what ways does it enhance or hinder your job performance?

Comparing the pros and cons side by side can assist you in determining whether it's useful to change this pattern of thinking. I've found that writing them down has helped me and my patients visualize how unnecessary it is to bring ourselves down constantly.

Gathering Evidence

In cognitive restructuring, a critical component is gathering evidence to support or challenge your thoughts and beliefs. This involves tracking triggering events, the individuals involved, and the activities. In addition, it can be helpful to note the intensity of your emotional responses and the memories that arise in connection with those events.

Gathering evidence involves examining the validity of your beliefs, assumptions, and thoughts. Cognitive distortions are often inaccurate and biased, yet they can be deeply ingrained. Overcoming these distortions requires gathering evidence that evaluates their rationality.

Therefore, it may be required to compile a list of factual information that attests to the truth of a belief and then compare it with evidence that shows the belief to be distorted or entirely false.

For instance, if you tend to personalize the actions of others and consistently blame yourself for things that are not your responsibility, it can be beneficial to gather evidence indicating that specific actions have no connection to you whatsoever. Then, by objectively examining the facts, you can challenge the distorted belief and gain a more accurate perspective.

Socratic Questioning

An integral aspect of cognitive restructuring involves developing the skill to question our thoughts and assumptions, particularly those that hinder our ability to lead productive lives. We have learnt in Chapter 5 that socratic questioning helps you ask questions that promote self-reflection and initiate problem-solving.

Adding to the examples of socratic questioning listed in Chapter 5, some insightful questions to ask yourself include:

- Is this situation truly black-and-white, or are there shades of gray?

- Is this thought driven by emotions or supported by factual evidence?

- Are there alternative interpretations or perspectives to consider?

- What evidence exists to validate this thought?

- What is the worst possible outcome, and how could I effectively respond?

- What evidence contradicts or challenges this thought?

- How can I test the validity of this belief?

For instance, if you find yourself engaging in catastrophizing, where you tend to assume the worst possible outcome in stressful situations, questioning this thought pattern can be helpful. First, create a list of all possible outcomes and assess the likelihood of each one.

By questioning, you open yourself up to alternative possibilities less extreme than the catastrophic scenarios you fear. This process allows for a more balanced and realistic perspective, ultimately reducing anxiety and promoting healthier thinking patterns.

Self-Monitoring

Identifying the underlying errors is crucial to transform an unproductive thought pattern. The effectiveness of cognitive restructuring relies on your ability to recognize the thoughts that trigger negative emotions and mental states.

Additionally, being mindful of when and where these thoughts arise can be beneficial. Certain situations may make you more susceptible to cognitive distortions, and being aware of these can help you proactively prepare.

For example, if you often experience self-doubt and negative self-talk when speaking in public, you might notice a distorted thinking pattern during presentations or meetings. Recognizing this vulnerability allows you to catch and modify negative thought before it undermines your confidence.

Engaging in self-reflection and observation can aid in this process. In addition, being mindful of your emotions and thoughts in different situations can help you identify patterns and triggers that cause negative thinking.

Through consistent self-monitoring, you will likely develop the ability to identify distorted thought patterns as they arise swiftly. This heightened awareness empowers you to intervene and engage in cognitive restructuring more effectively.

Thought Record

Keeping thought records has been a game changer for many of my patients. It has the ability to heighten your awareness of previously unquestioned or unnoticed cognitive distortions, marking a crucial initial step toward restructuring them.

There are various approaches to structuring a thought record, but the fundamental concept involves documenting recurring thoughts and the corresponding situations in which they arise. One commonly used thought record prompts you to record the situation, thoughts, emotions, behaviors, and alternate thoughts.

Let's consider a couple of examples to illustrate this process. First, suppose you often experience social anxiety and tend to catastrophize social interactions. In that case, you might complete the thought record as follows:

- Situation: Attending a social gathering with unfamiliar people.

- Thoughts: Everyone is going to judge me and think I'm boring. I'll embarrass myself.

- Emotions: Anxiety, self-consciousness.

- Behaviors: Avoid attending the event, isolate myself.

- Alternate thought: It's normal to feel nervous in new social situations. People are generally friendly and understanding. I can focus on being myself and engaging in conversation.

Alternatively, if you struggle with low self-esteem and negative self-perception, your thought record may appear as follows:

- Situation: Receiving constructive criticism at work.

- Thoughts: I'm a failure. I'm never good enough. I'll never succeed.

- Emotions: Sadness, frustration.

- Behaviors: Dwelled on self-critical thoughts, become demotivated.

- Alternate thought: Constructive criticism is an opportunity for growth and improvement. I can learn from feedback and strive to enhance my skills.

By committing these details to writing, you can gain a valuable tool to explore previously unnoticed aspects and identify thought patterns that may indicate specific cognitive distortions.

Decatastrophizing

Essentially, this approach involves asking yourself, "What is the worst-case scenario?" and thoroughly examining all possible consequences. Frequently, we find ourselves burdened with anxieties or assumptions about the most extreme and unlikely repercussions, even if they would not have a catastrophic impact on our lives.

Decatastrophizing, or engaging in "what if?" thinking, allows you to evaluate the likelihood of different outcomes, alleviate irrational or unreasonable anxiety, and recognize that even in the worst-case scenario, the situation remains manageable. You can gain a more balanced perspective and regain control by challenging exaggerated fears.

Art Therapy and Core Wounds

We've delved into art therapy on Chapter 2 of this book. However, it's important to note that art therapy plays a significant role in healing core wounds resulting from childhood trauma, as it provides a unique and practical approach to addressing these wounds and facilitating healing. Through this creative process, you can access and express emotions, memories, and experiences related to your childhood trauma in a non-verbal and symbolic manner.

Art therapy offers control and empowerment if you have felt powerless during your traumatic experiences. The creative process allows individuals the freedom to express their agency, make decisions, and create narratives that redefine their perception of their traumatic history. By engaging in art-making and witnessing the transformation of your artwork, you can experience a sense of accomplishment, resilience, and hope.

Mindfulness Techniques for Emotional Regulation

Throughout the day, we all experience a wide range of emotions that naturally arise and fade away, regardless of whether we consciously allow them to do so. However, when we develop the skill of mindfulness and cultivate the ability to sit with our emotions, even the uncomfortable ones, we gain the capacity to manage them effectively.

Practicing mindfulness of emotions involves acknowledging them without judgment, which allows us to grow and evolve as individuals. Rather than pushing feelings away, we learn to engage with them, leading to personal development. Conversely, neglecting our emotions for an extended period can hinder our personal growth and diminish our presence for those we care about.

By embracing the practice of mindfulness, specifically towards our emotions, we can enhance our ability to regulate emotional reactivity. Through consistent practice, we can achieve a state of greater mental calmness. Some approaches to cultivating mindfulness of emotions and integrating it into our daily lives include practicing self-acceptance, observing your feelings, mindfulness-based cognitive therapy, and meditation.

Practicing Self-Acceptance

The primary lesson to derive from practicing mindfulness is the importance of self-acceptance. Recognizing that you don't need to become someone else or strive for perfection is essential. Understanding that imperfection is a natural part of being human is crucial.

This doesn't imply that you can't pursue positive transformations in your life. However, in the present moment, accepting yourself for who you are equips you with the necessary tools to navigate your daily emotions and foster a healthier state of being.

Observing Your Feelings

Instead of trying to decipher the future implications or the origins of your feelings, simply observe them in the present moment. Avoid engaging in interpretations about what your emotions might signify or how your thoughts came to be. For instance, when thoughts such as "I'm not good enough for this opportunity" or "I'll never succeed in this endeavor" arise, recognize them as mere thoughts without attaching any immediate significance.

I often tell my patients who tend to overanalyze their thoughts: how you want to respond to your thoughts is up to you. You can disregard them, hoping they will fade away, or you can analyze them and potentially intensify your anxiety. However, ultimately, the best option is to acknowledge that the thought has emerged and allow it to exist without taking immediate action.

You're not obligated to act based on these fleeting feelings. It's important to let your emotions exist without letting them define you. Instead, concentrate on making progress toward your goals. Giving yourself enough time to reflect on the reasons behind your negative thoughts is essential. However, waiting until you feel ready to tackle this task is best.

Meditation

There's growing evidence that mindfulness meditation is effective in managing emotions. The National Center for Complementary and Integrative Health states that consistent meditation can enhance mental well-being (Meditation and Mindfulness: What You Need to Know, 2022).

As someone who frequently meditates and has seen the positive results of meditation in my patients, I can't recommend it enough. Regular meditation provides many benefits, including improved management of stress, depression, anxiety, sleep, concentration, and substance use. Meditation is a beneficial practice that requires no tools, props, or financial investment. This ensures that anyone can access it at any time, from anywhere.

Journaling Exercises for Identifying Triggers and Emotions

During my childhood, one of the few places I could find solace was in the pages of my diary. Little did I know that it's a prevalent activity often prescribed to patients in the field of psychology and that years later, I would be recommending it to my own patients.

Journaling is a readily available and low-demand tool for effectively managing your emotions. Putting your thoughts and feelings into writing can assist in addressing various emotional hurdles that may impede your progress. Incorporating journaling into your daily routine can promote emotional well-being and enhance overall mental health. Maintaining a personal space where you can freely express and delve into your inner thoughts allows you to gain valuable perspectives and better understand your needs and desires.

If facing a blank page seems overwhelming, utilizing prompts can offer valuable support and guidance to kickstart your journaling practice. In this section, I'll provide various prompts for emotional healing, emotional security, self-compassion, and emotional awareness that I've found to be beneficial for myself and my patients.

Emotional Healing Prompts

Navigating the lingering effects of a challenging childhood can pose significant challenges. Journaling can be a valuable tool for processing emotions, fostering healing, and self-discovery. Here are some prompts to aid you in your emotional healing:

1. Reflect on a specific childhood memory that still holds emotional weight for you. Describe the emotions associated with it and how it has influenced your life.

2. Write a letter to your younger self, offering comfort, understanding, and encouragement.

3. Identify three core values that are important to you and explore how your childhood experiences have shaped them.

4. Describe a positive role model or mentor you wish to have during childhood. How would their presence have impacted your life?

5. Write about a challenging emotion or recurring pattern you want to overcome. Explore its origins and brainstorm strategies for addressing and transforming it.

6. List three things you appreciate about yourself and your journey of resilience.

7. Describe an activity or hobby that brings you joy and allows you to reconnect with your authentic self. Write about how engaging in this activity makes you feel.

8. Reflect on a moment of self-compassion and kindness you have shown yourself recently. How did it make you feel, and how can you continue cultivating self-compassion moving forward?

9. Write about a boundary or limit you would like to set to protect your emotional well-being. Explore why it's essential and how you can communicate it effectively.

10. Imagine your ideal future self, free from the burdens of your difficult childhood. Describe this version of yourself and the steps you can take to move closer to embodying that vision.

Emotional Security Prompts

Attachment theory posits that infants establish varying bonds with their primary caregivers, and the quality of these bonds relies on the caregiver's responsiveness to the baby's needs. Children who form secure attachments generally meet their needs consistently, fostering their ability to cultivate and maintain healthy relationships as adults.

On the other hand, children who experience inconsistent responses to their needs are more prone to developing anxious attachments in their relationships with others. Research indicates that individuals struggling to form secure emotional bonds with their caregivers may encounter difficulties in adult relationships (Fleck et al., 2017).

If you find it challenging to establish emotional security in your relationships, you may want to engage in the following journal prompts with your partner, friends, or family members as a means of support:

1. How can we establish healthy boundaries in our relationship to promote feelings of safety and security?

2. What are my individual needs within this relationship? How can we navigate them together?

3. What actions or behaviors from my partner, friend, or family member would help me feel that my needs are being met?

4. How can we enhance communication to better understand and support each other's emotional needs?

5. Reflect on a past relationship where you felt emotionally secure. What were the factors or dynamics that contributed to that sense of security? How can we incorporate those elements into our current relationship?

6. Identify any patterns or triggers that evoke feelings of insecurity or anxiety in our relationship. How can we address and navigate these triggers together?

7. How can we foster a sense of emotional safety and trust within our relationship? Are there any past experiences or wounds that need healing or addressing?

Self-Compassion Prompts

If you often find it challenging to extend self-compassion, even in the presence of supportive individuals, it may be beneficial to focus on nurturing a kinder relationship with yourself. Self-judgment, often fueled by cognitive distortions, can hinder the practice of self-compassion.

Cognitive distortions involve distorted or biased thoughts that tend to amplify negativity. To cultivate self-compassion, Neidich recommends engaging with the following writing prompts:

1. What underlying purpose or intention does being hard on myself serve? How does it impact my well-being?

2. In this present moment, what would it take for me to show greater kindness and gentleness towards myself?

3. Imagine yourself speaking to a small child who needs comfort and reassurance. How would you communicate with them? How can you extend the same tone of compassion and understanding to yourself?

4. Reflect on a recent situation where you were overly critical or judgmental towards yourself. What alternative perspective or compassionate response could have been more helpful and supportive?

5. What affirming and nurturing statements can I remind myself of during challenging times?

6. Identify any recurring self-defeating thoughts or beliefs that contribute to self-judgment. How can I challenge or reframe these thoughts to promote self-compassion?

7. How can I prioritize self-care and self-compassion in my daily routine? What specific actions or practices can I incorporate to cultivate a more compassionate mindset?

Emotional Awareness Prompts

Developing emotional awareness is a crucial step in recognizing and identifying the emotions you're experiencing. If you find yourself unsure about the specific emotions of anger, sadness, or disappointment, utilizing prompts can aid in uncovering and processing these feelings effectively.

Many individuals may encounter emotional challenges because they mask or avoid acknowledging their genuine emotions. However, when we confront our emotions directly and allow ourselves to sit with them, the distress often diminishes, leading to a greater sense of emotional well-being.

Delving into the core of your feelings can also provide valuable insights into your emotional landscape and how these emotions impact your life. To assist you in processing your feelings, try the following initial journal prompts.

1. What emotions arise when I reflect on recent challenging situations or interactions?

2. Are there any recurring patterns or themes in my emotions that I've noticed?

3. How does my body physically respond when I experience certain emotions? Are there any sensations or tension I can identify?

4. Are there any underlying beliefs or thoughts that contribute to the intensity or duration of my emotions?

5. Are there any past experiences or unresolved issues that might influence my emotional state?

6. How do I typically express or suppress my emotions? Are there healthier ways I could approach them?

7. How do my emotions affect my daily life, relationships, and overall well-being?

8. What self-care practices or activities comfort me and help me regulate my emotions?

9. Can I identify any triggers or specific situations that evoke strong emotional responses?

10. How can I cultivate a compassionate and understanding attitude toward myself when experiencing difficult emotions?

'Reparent your inner child with tenderness, for their journey shapes the landscape of your soul.'

Louise Hay

———

CHAPTER 8

Reparenting Inner Child

C hildren who grow up in households characterized by trauma and dysfunction often face difficulties acquiring boundaries and behaviors that many others consider natural. As children observe and learn from their caregivers, they internalize their examples of interaction with the world. If these caregivers exhibit dysfunctional or unhealthy behaviors, children are likely to imitate them, even unintentionally.

Reflecting on our childhood and adolescent experiences often unveils insights into adult behavior. The interactions we have with our caregivers and their interactions with each other shape our perception of the world and those around us. Consequently, our sense of self, communication style, and ability to form relationships are profoundly influenced. We must cultivate self-awareness and actively work on our behaviors to avoid repeating these patterns throughout adulthood.

Needing a Lot of Time and Space to Yourself

Experiencing a tumultuous or unstable upbringing can significantly affect your health and happiness. The constant stress from such circumstances leaves your central nervous system in constant hypervigilance. As a result, you may need ample time alone to calm the symptoms of anxiety, nervousness, and fear that lingers within you.

Being in your own home provides a feeling of safety and comfort because you're in a familiar environment you can manage. However, in more extreme cases, you might even notice traits of agoraphobia or social anxiety. Recognizing these patterns and seeking support to overcome their challenges is essential.

Serial Monogamy

Many of my patients report engaging in serial monogamy when we begin our sessions. This results from underlying fears stemming from past hurts, the fear of loneliness, or the desire to validate the worthiness of love and affection they didn't experience in their childhood. Each new partner represents an opportunity to seek confirmation and fulfillment, hoping to find the love and companionship that may have been absent in their past experiences.

Abandonment Issues

If you've endured neglect or abandonment in your childhood, the impact can extend into adulthood, manifesting as lingering fears of being left behind. Even if you may not consciously recognize these fears on the surface, they can subtly influence your thoughts and actions.

Although the underlying fear revolves around the possibility of your partner, friend, or family member leaving, these anxieties often surface in mundane scenarios. For example, during my own adolescence, I often felt anxious when my partner would go out alone or when they temporarily stepped away during an argument.

Some of my patients' abandonment issues manifest as jealousy and, in more severe cases, possessiveness as they strive to maintain a sense of security and control in their relationships. Acknowledging and addressing your fears is crucial because they can significantly affect the quality of your relationships and overall well-being.

Trying to Change People

This reaction to trauma comes from the thought that we must maximize what we currently possess, or from the anxiety that we may never acquire anything better. As a child, we were powerless to change our caregivers, so we adapted by trying to make the best of the situation. As adults, it's common for this pattern to carry over into our relationships, leading us to seek changes within our partners, friends, and family to alleviate our relationship-related fears. The underlying desire is to "fix" the people in our lives and transform them into better versions, ultimately proving to ourselves that we deserve and are capable of fulfilling relationships.

Experiencing Irritability or Being Easily Annoyed by Others

When raised in environments characterized by frequent criticism or observing others being criticized, we internalize this as the standard way to express dissatisfaction within relationships. We start believing our flaws and quirks are unacceptable, so we tend to project this intolerance onto our partners, friends, and family.

Unequal Household and Financial Responsibilities

At times, this behavior can manifest as a hesitancy to rely on anyone, stemming from fears of dependence on someone else. In other instances, it can manifest as assuming complete financial and/or household responsibilities within the partnership or excessively caring for the other person to the extent of being taken advantage of. On the contrary, relying overly on your partner, friends, or family to the point where they assume full caretaking responsibilities is also a consequence of unmet childhood needs.

Remaining in Dead-End Relationships

Growing up in unstable environments, where caregivers grapple with mental illness, drug addiction, or even illness and death, can instill a sense of guilt in children. This guilt arises from a desire to end a relationship before being able to "fix" the other person. Sometimes, staying with someone who isn't a suitable match might feel safer than being alone.

Lingering Uncertainty

The pervasive sense of uncertainty you experience in various aspects of life can be attributed to caregivers who were unreliable or abandoned you, instilling a deep-seated distrust of those who claim to care for you. If you harbor the fear of being hurt by others in a similar manner as your caregivers, the inclination to avoid settling down can provide a perceived sense of safety. It allows you to exit the relationship when necessary, empowering you to protect yourself.

Persistently Fighting or Consistently Avoiding Confrontation in Relationships

In relationships, conflict is a natural occurrence. Yet, if you were exposed to constant arguments between caregivers or grew up in conflict-avoidant environments, you may need to acquire the essential skills for effective and healthy communication. Consequently, you may need more tools to navigate and manage conflict productively. This includes developing healthy strategies to address and resolve conflicts constructively and positively.

Limited Knowledge of How to Make Amends

As highlighted in the previous point, the absence of learning effective strategies for managing conflict healthily also affects our ability to repair relationships following inevitable disputes that arise in partnerships. Consequently, we may exhibit behaviors such as pretending the conflict didn't occur, struggling to identify when or how to compromise on an issue, or resorting to giving the silent treatment. These patterns reflect our limited understanding of how to address and heal relationship wounds, hindering the process of repairing and strengthening the bond with our partners, friends, and family.

Developing Self-Love and Self-Compassion

What Is Self-Love and Self-Compassion?

Self-compassion and self-love are closely intertwined yet distinct concepts. Practicing self-compassion means being kind and understanding towards yourself when facing personal failures or difficulties. It means extending the same compassion to oneself as one would to a cherished friend—acknowledging your suffering, empathizing with you, and offering kindness and understanding.

On the other hand, self-love encompasses an overall appreciation and regard for oneself, nurtured through actions that promote physical, psychological, and spiritual growth. It revolves around recognizing one's worth as a human deserving of love and respect.

While self-compassion can be accessed at any moment, self-love is a more enduring state that requires intentional cultivation over time. It involves building a foundation of self-value and self-care to foster a lasting sense of self-appreciation and acceptance.

How to Cultivate Self-Love

When I mention self-love to my older patients for the first time, they often think it's some modern notion and dismiss it as self-indulgence. They mistakenly associate self-love with self-centeredness and equate it to narcissism, a trait many have reported their parents having.

However, self-love is not about fostering an inflated ego or a sense of superiority. Instead, it entails attending to your needs and acknowledging your inherent worth. Self-love is a compassionate practice emphasizing self-care and self-acceptance, recognizing that you deserve kindness and nurturing. It's a vital aspect of personal growth and well-being.

Our relationship with ourselves is crucial as it sets the foundation for interacting with others. Prioritizing self-love allows us to live in harmony with our values and make positive choices in our daily lives. Confidence, self-respect, self-worth, and self-love are interconnected facets of our being that mutually influence and shape one another. As we nurture and strengthen our love for ourselves, it also deepens the love we can give and receive from others. By fostering a solid foundation of self-love, we can cultivate more fulfilling and meaningful relationships with those around us.

At times, asserting oneself and prioritizing personal needs can be challenging. While sporadic acts of self-love may be considerate, embracing it as a daily practice is crucial. Here are some ways to integrate self-love into your lifestyle:

Prioritize Your Mental Health and Well-Being

It's crucial to understand the correlation between your physical and mental well-being. Your physical well-being can significantly affect your mental and emotional state. When you prioritize and nurture your body, you also positively influence your mental health. Maintaining a nutritious diet and ensuring sufficient sleep are crucial for your physical health and overall well-being. These practices can also help prevent illnesses.

Change a Negative Mindset

Positive thinking goes beyond simply disregarding problems; it involves adopting a positive outlook on life that encompasses gratitude and recognizing numerous possibilities. As part of this mindset, seeking support in processing anger, releasing resentment, and letting go of grudges may be beneficial.

Holding onto and fixating on anger and hatred toward others can harm our mental and emotional well-being. Addressing these negative emotions at their root cause can be an act of self-love and self-care.

Speaking kind words to yourself is crucial. Positive affirmations have the power to enhance self-esteem and alleviate social fears. Remind yourself that you're a compassionate individual doing your best. Shifting your perspective and focusing on aspects you're grateful for and appreciate can bring immense uplifting and serve as another means of practicing self-love.

Avoid Comparing Yourself to Other People

When we see someone achieving great success in their career while we feel stuck in our jobs, or when we compare our appearance to that of celebrities or models and feel dissatisfied with ourselves, it's natural to feel down. Social comparisons can be a significant source of stress, triggering emotions such as anxiety, self-doubt, and discontentment. While healthy competition and comparison can sometimes be motivating, more often than not, they have a diminishing effect, leading to negative emotions like stress, guilt, and shame.

The rise of social media has profoundly impacted our mental health, and not always in a positive way. It has intensified our tendency to judge ourselves harshly, constantly comparing our lives, achievements, and appearance to others. This constant self-evaluation leaves us feeling inadequate and fosters a sense of not being good enough. Studies have also shown that excessive use of social media is associated with higher rates of depression and other mental health issues.

Surround Yourself With Loving, Supportive People

It's essential to have a reliable support system for our overall well-being. Most people's parents and siblings are a foundational part of their support system. However, familial relationships may be strained or unavailable for people who've had a traumatic childhood at the hands of their family. In such cases, it becomes essential to cultivate relationships with friends and community members who can provide care and support.

Letting go of toxic and draining friendships that don't contribute to your growth and well-being is vital. Instead, focus on nurturing connections with individuals who believe in you, uplift you, and support your journey of self-discovery and personal growth.

In romantic relationships, it is fundamental to seek deep emotional connections and intimacy. Invest your time, energy, and care into romantic and platonic relationships that bring you joy, energize you, and provide a sense of restoration. These healthy relationships will support you in becoming the best version of yourself.

Forgive Yourself

It's crucial to develop strategies to overcome self-loathing in all its forms. Try to forgive yourself and embrace healing as a means of incorporating self-love into your daily life. Instead of dwelling on past mistakes and regrets, avoid dwelling on them. Instead of blaming yourself for circumstances that may have been beyond your control, shift your focus towards self-forgiveness.

One study found that cultivating forgiveness is associated with reduced stress and a decrease in symptoms related to mental health (Shields et al., 2016). By embracing self-forgiveness, you can foster a healthier mindset and enhance your overall well-being.

Set Boundaries

Establishing boundaries is a valuable tool for managing stress. It's essential to assert yourself and learn to say "no" when necessary, professionally or personally, to protect your energy and well-being. One-sided relationships, characterized by an imbalance in energy, control, and consideration, can be draining and unsustainable. Acknowledging your needs and allocating dedicated time to prioritize self-care by setting clear boundaries is crucial. This practice allows you to be mindful of your well-being and maintain a healthy balance in your interactions and commitments.

How to Practice Self-Compassion

Showing compassion and support to a friend or loved one during difficult times usually comes naturally. We offer them understanding, hope, guidance, and encouragement. However, when we encounter our own challenges, we tend to be more self-critical and harsh. We scrutinize our thoughts and actions, leading to feelings of unworthiness, shame, and frustration.

In our eagerness to progress, we might use phrases like "stop being so sensitive" or "don't let it affect you" to minimize our emotions. Although these intentions are meant to help us navigate emotional struggles, they can generate excessive stress and become significant barriers to experiencing happiness within ourselves and our relationships with others. Fortunately, several methods can assist you in overcoming these obstacles and promoting self-compassion.

Care for Yourself

We sometimes prioritize caring for others and neglect or disregard our own needs. However, when we embrace self-compassion, we acknowledge that we also have needs that deserve to be fulfilled, and we deserve to engage in self-care activities. By establishing self-care practices, we can reduce the inclination to resort to unhealthy coping mechanisms when confronted with challenges and stress.

Consider How You'd Talk to a Friend

We often offer our friends and loved ones kind words, hope, and encouragement. The next time you encounter a problematic situation, consider how you would advise a close friend experiencing something similar.

Become an Observer

When we come across emotional challenges or difficult moments, we often seem caught up in reactive survival mode. However, by intentionally slowing down and creating some space, we can step back and observe our experience more objectively. This broader perspective allows us to maintain a sense of perspective and gain valuable insights that might have otherwise gone unnoticed. By pausing and observing, we empower ourselves to navigate challenging situations with greater awareness and make more informed choices.

Change Your Self-Talk

Become aware of your inner dialogue during moments of negative emotions. Pay attention to how you speak to yourself, and consciously change negative self-talk into more encouraging and positive language. Aim for a voice that resembles that of a supportive mentor or advocate rather than a harsh critic or judge. By adopting this new approach to self-talk, you can cultivate a more compassionate and encouraging mindset that promotes self-growth and emotional well-being.

Be Clear About What You Want

By actively working on reframing critical thoughts into nurturing self-talk, you can begin to unravel insights into your desires and needs. Pause momentarily and reflect on what you truly want, need, and yearn for. Clarifying these needs will enable you to focus on your aspirations and goals, boosting your motivation and overall fulfillment.

Keep a Journal and Write It Out

In the previous chapters of this book, I've highlighted the significance of journaling at length. However, it's also important to stress its role in practicing self-compassion. When journaling with self-compassion, remember instances where your thoughts tend to veer into critical statements or when you start to feel isolated in your experiences. Just as you would with self-talk, purposefully reframe any critical comments using a gentler and more empathetic tone to explore how it can create a different emotional response. By engaging in this reflective practice, you can cultivate greater self-awareness and potentially discover alternative perspectives that promote self-compassion and understanding.

Cognitive Behavioral Therapy Techniques for Challenging Negative Self-Talk

Automatic Negative Thinking

In prior chapters, we have learnt that CBT can help in overcoming anxiety and panic attacks. However, when it comes to reparenting yourself, CBT can be used to challenge negative self-talk.

Negative self-talk is often the result of automatic negative thoughts (ANTs), which encompass the spontaneous thoughts that arise from our deeply ingrained beliefs about ourselves and the world. These thoughts emerge effortlessly and unconsciously, serving as the running commentary of our stream of consciousness. They can manifest as descriptions, inferences, or evaluations directly linked to specific situations, often occurring without deliberate control or intention.

As their name suggests, automatic thoughts are not under direct control, as they arise as reflexive reactions rooted in our beliefs about ourselves and the world. However, it's possible to indirectly influence these thoughts by challenging the underlying assumptions that give rise to them. By addressing and questioning these beliefs, you can effectively control the automatic ideas you generate.

Methods to Combat Negative Self-Talk and Automatic Thoughts

Thought/Feeling Record

This first exercise aims to address negative automatic thoughts in a targeted manner, one by one, by exploring their triggers and consequences. By engaging in this exercise, you can better understand their negative automatic thoughts and learn how to replace them with more positive ones. It's particularly beneficial if you're seeking to examine your thought patterns thoroughly.

Recognizing distorted thinking patterns within ourselves can be challenging and distressing. However, I've witnessed many of my patients identify, comprehend, and rectify faulty thinking patterns by following these instructions whenever a negative automatic thought pops up:

1. Write down the date and time of the situation that caused the negative automatic thought.

2. Describe the situation, reflecting on the factors that led to this event and the unpleasant emotions you're experiencing.

3. Document the ANTs that emerged during this situation. Take note of the specific thoughts and images that came up, and assess your belief level on a scale from 1 (no belief at all) to 10 (complete belief).

4. Identify the emotions that accompanied your thoughts and images. Emotions are often wordless experiences, while thoughts have a more structured nature. Rate the intensity of each emotion on a scale from 1 (barely felt) to 10 (overwhelming).

5. Explore your response to the situation. Recognize any cognitive distortions or faulty thinking styles that you employed at the time. Consider your worst-case scenario in this situation and assess the

likelihood of it occurring on a scale from 1 (not likely at all) to 10 (extremely likely).

6. Develop a more adaptive response to challenge your automatic thoughts. Gather evidence that supports or refutes your automatic thoughts, and consider alternative outcomes. Counter the worst-case scenario by envisioning a best-case scenario, then aim for a "most realistic" scenario. Rate the likelihood of the most realistic scenario on a scale from 1 (not likely at all) to 10 (extremely likely).

7. Reflect on the outcome of the event. Assess whether your feelings have changed after challenging your automatic thoughts. Consider the degree of belief you have in your automatic thoughts now, and whether you're more inclined to consider positive or realistic scenarios. Compare how you felt before and now, and rate the intensity of your automatic thoughts at this point.

Challenging Thoughts With Questions

This exercise consists of a carefully crafted set of questions designed to challenge automatic thoughts. It's a valuable resource for disputing negative thoughts and complements the above mentioned exercises. With its straightforward approach, this exercise is an excellent choice if you wish to incorporate Socratic questioning and fact-checking techniques into addressing ANTs. Additionally, it offers a convenient and accessible resource that can effectively help individuals deal with such thoughts.

Below is a compilation of questions designed to challenge automatic thoughts:

1. How have I dealt with similar situations in the past? What strategies or coping mechanisms have worked for me before?

2. What evidence or facts support this thought? Is there any existing evidence or experiences that contradict it?

3. Besides myself, what other external factors or circumstances might be influencing this situation? How can I consider these factors?

4. If I sought advice from a counselor or therapist, what guidance would they provide for this situation?

5. What aspects of this event or person am I ready to accept? What can I realistically control, and what should I let go of?

6. Will this thought and its impact matter in the long run? How significant will it be in a day, a week, or a month from now?

7. Am I overgeneralizing based on experience? Is this thought applicable to the current situation?

8. Do I have genuine control over the factors related to this thought? What aspects are within my sphere of influence?

9. If this thought were true, what would be the worst possible outcome? Is it a realistic or exaggerated view?

10. Are my thoughts helping me effectively deal with this scenario, or are they adding to the difficulty or distress?

11. Is there a positive or alternative perspective I can take on this thought? Are there any silver linings or potential growth opportunities?

12. What advice would I give a close friend facing a similar scenario? How can I extend the same kindness and guidance to myself?

13. Am I using rigid and inflexible thinking patterns such as "I must," "I have to," or "I should"? Are these thoughts necessary and realistic?

Getting Rid of ANTs

This straightforward exercise begins by providing information about automatic thoughts and their impact. It then guides you through the process of identifying your triggers, ANTs, and adaptive views to help you comprehend and, if needed, challenge your automatic thoughts.

Frequently, ANTs are triggered by specific environmental factors, such as our interactions or life events. You can identify and address these triggers by working through the table below, from left to right. In the first column, list some of your common triggers. In the center column, jot down the corresponding ANT that tends to arise with each trigger. Finally, in the right-hand column, challenge yourself to develop a more positive, constructive, self-compassionate, and helpful thought that can replace the ANT.

For example:

Trigger	ANT	Adaptive Thought
E.g. Failing a test.	"I'm never going to graduate and have a successful career."	"I didn't study enough, but that's okay. Next time, I'm going to begin studying a week before the test and ace it."

Challenging Different Types of ANTs

This last exercise comprehensively explores ten specific types of ANTs and how they appear in various everyday scenarios. By engaging in this exercise, you can identify each kind of ANT more effectively, leading to a greater understanding of your subconscious thought patterns and paving the way for their replacement.

The table below examines ten distinct types of ANTs. In the rightmost column, try to create an example for each ANT. Possible examples are given in the third column; now it's your turn to provide your own examples in the final column.

Type	Description	Example #1	Example #2
Selective Abstraction	Drawing broad conclusions about an entire situation based on a single or minor negative attribute.	"I made a small mistake in my presentation, so I must be a terrible public speaker."	
All-or-Nothing Reasoning	Seeing things in strictly black-and-white terms, neglecting the potential for shades of gray or varying degrees of possibility.	"Either I'm a complete success or a total failure in life."	
Emotional Reasoning	Using personal emotions as justification for one's thoughts or beliefs.	"I feel anxious about going to the party, so it must mean that something bad will happen there."	
Arbitrary Inference	Making judgments or reaching conclusions without having access to all the necessary information or facts.	"I didn't receive a reply to my text message, so they must be mad at me."	
Moral Imperatives	Applying rigid and inflexible standards to	"It's not okay to change your mind, ever."	

	oneself, others, and various aspects of life.		
Minimization/ Magnification	Exaggerating or magnifying the negative aspects of a situation while minimizing or downplaying the positive aspects.	"The dinner wasn't good because I forgot to put enough salt in the dish."	
Global Judgments	Assigning derogatory or negative labels to isolated events or individuals.	"I'm completely incompetent at my job."	
Personalization	Taking personal responsibility for circumstances or events that are outside your control.	"It's my fault that my parents are fighting."	
Overgeneralizat ion	Making sweeping generalizations based on isolated incidents, using one event to form judgments about all other similar events.	"I dropped something, because I'm a klutz."	

Discounting the Positive	Focusing on the negatives in positive situations or events, or interpreting positive outcomes as negative ones.	"They're only saying that to get your vote."	

Acceptance and Commitment Therapy Technique

Acceptance and Commitment Therapy (ACT) and Mindfulness-Based Cognitive Therapy (MBCT) synergistically offer a powerful treatment approach. By integrating mindfulness skills and self-acceptance, ACT promotes the acceptance of thoughts and feelings without struggle or guilt. This combined approach is effective in addressing various medical conditions such as Obsessive-Compulsive Disorder (OCD), depression, anxiety, and substance abuse.

ACT emphasizes the importance of commitment in cultivating acceptance. Rather than avoiding or evading stressful situations, ACT encourages facing challenges directly. It involves committing to actions that foster personal growth and embracing the difficulties that arise. This approach not only treats psychological disorders, but also empowers you to take charge of your life and make choices aligned with your values.

Two essential processes in ACT, cognitive fusion/defusion and experiential avoidance, significantly impact our psychological well-being. Understanding these processes is crucial in ACT, as they can hinder psychological flexibility and prevent us from living in alignment with our values. By exploring fusion/defusion and experiential avoidance, we can gain insights into their impact and learn effective strategies to cultivate mindfulness, self-acceptance, and compassionate responses to our thoughts and emotions.

Fusion/Defusion

Cognitive fusion in ACT is the attachment to thoughts that control our behavior and contribute to emotional distress. Fusion limits our flexibility and hinders us from pursuing meaningful goals. ACT uses mindfulness to promote defusion and psychological flexibility, allowing us to observe thoughts without judgment. By practicing "noticing and naming" our thoughts, we create distance and recognize them as passing mental events. This empowers us to approach thoughts with curiosity and openness. ACT emphasizes taking purposeful action and cultivating self-compassion to counteract emotional pain and self-defeating behaviors. Regular practice of self-compassion strengthens connections, prioritizes values, and supports committed action.

Experiential Avoidance

Experiential avoidance, a defense mechanism employed when confronted with emotionally unpleasant or anxiety-inducing situations, offers us an escape route when we perceive danger. Paradoxically, this form of avoidance sustains distress and amplifies and intensifies it. Engaging in avoidance to evade challenging thoughts and emotions is counterproductive and runs contrary to self-compassion. In ACT, instead of avoiding them, we consciously acknowledge and embrace these emotions without passing judgment. By cultivating curiosity and non-attachment, we prevent these thoughts and feelings from exerting excessive control over our lives.

Embracing the reality of our circumstances with kindness and compassion enables us to respond with greater flexibility and alignment to our deeply held values—our aspirations and principles. In the ACT model, "acceptance" is an active commitment to taking purposeful action that enriches our potential for a meaningful and fulfilling life.

How to Practice Acceptance and Commitment Therapy

ACT offers a transformative approach to enhancing mental well-being and living more meaningfully. By incorporating ACT techniques, individuals can develop psychological flexibility, cultivate self-compassion, and embrace their thoughts and feelings without judgment. ACT encourages a shift from struggling against unwanted experiences to accepting them as part of the human experience. It allows individuals to make choices aligned with their values and take committed action. Through mindfulness, acceptance, and values-based living, ACT empowers individuals to overcome psychological challenges and foster personal growth.

Below are some approaches to cultivating self-compassion through ACT:

1. Practice mindfulness: Mindfulness is a core component of ACT and can enhance self-compassion. By being present and non-judgmentally aware of your thoughts, emotions, and sensations, you can cultivate self-compassion in the face of challenging experiences.

2. Defusion exercises: Engage in defusion techniques to create distance from your negative thoughts and self-critical judgments. Recognize that thoughts are merely mental events and not necessarily accurate reflections of reality. Use strategies like "noticing and naming" your thoughts to reduce their impact and promote self-compassion.

3. Cultivate self-acceptance: Embrace your thoughts and emotions without judgment or resistance. Acceptance involves acknowledging and allowing these experiences to arise without trying to change or suppress them. By accepting yourself as you are, you create space for self-compassion to flourish.

4. Connect with values: Clarify your core values—what truly matters to you—and align your actions with them. Even while experiencing difficult emotions, engaging in value-driven behaviors can foster self-compassion by reinforcing your commitment to living by your values.

5. Engage in self-care: Prioritize activities promoting physical, emotional, and mental well-being. Treat yourself with kindness, compassion, and understanding. Take breaks, engage in activities you enjoy, seek support from loved ones, and practice self-compassionate self-talk.

6. Seek therapy or group support: Consider working with an ACT therapist or joining a group focusing on self-compassion and mindfulness. Therapeutic guidance and the support of others can deepen your understanding of self-compassion and provide practical tools for its integration into your life.

'Release the chains of shame and guilt, and step into the freedom of self-acceptance.'

Brené Brown

———

CHAPTER 9

—

Release of shame and guilt

S hame and guilt are common self-conscious emotions that we experience throughout our lives. These emotions are often negative and can create discomfort.

When I began my healing journey, I found it difficult to determine whether I was experiencing shame or guilt, and I've seen many of my patients also struggle with it. However, understanding the distinction between these emotions and identifying the underlying cause of your feelings is essential in guiding us toward finding the most effective path for personal growth and moving forward.

What Is Shame?

Shame is a profound emotion linked to moral wrongdoing or reprehensible behavior that can be heightened when exposed. It can also attach itself to thoughts or actions that remain undisclosed. Shame enters our moral character when we measure our actions against ethical standards and realize that we fall short.

When we overlook our shortcomings, we can be made aware of them and experience shame. Conversely, if we are unfazed by being made aware of our shortcomings, we can be deemed shameless. Shame can also stem from a lack of honorable qualities shared by others, particularly if this absence is our own fault.

Common manifestations of shame I see in my patients include

- avoiding eye contact

- covering the brow and eyes

- adopting a slouched posture

- stuttering

- speaking in an overly soft voice

- crying

- experiencing warmth or heat

- being unable to move or feeling frozen

- mental confusion

While shame can lead to remorse and repentance and inspire forgiveness, it can also be regarded as embarrassing, prompting us to keep it hidden. But how does shame form in the first place?

Since birth, you have been learning to assess when and whether you're okay or if your environment accepts or rejects you, shaping your self-esteem through experiences of praise or criticism, discipline or punishment, and care or neglect. Unfortunately, if you grew up in an abusive environment, you're likely burdened with the belief that you're inferior, inadequate, and undeserving, leading to a pervasive sense of shame.

Over time, this intense shame can significantly impact your self-image and contribute to low self-esteem. Feelings of shame are often rooted in the opinions of others, causing you to become hypersensitive to perceived criticism and experience a sense of rejection. For many years, I harbored painful self-contempt and a feeling of worthlessness, and I witnessed it in many of my patients as well.

What Is Guilt?

Where shame centers around personal inadequacy, guilt is tied to specific actions and involves blame and remorse. It's important to note that shame often arises from not meeting societal moral standards, whereas guilt stems from falling short of one's ethical standards. As a result, we can experience guilt even for socially acceptable actions that contradict our values, such as living luxuriously or consuming animal products.

Shame and guilt frequently coexist, leading to confusion between the two. For example, when you harm someone, you may feel remorse for your actions (guilt) and a sense of personal worthlessness (shame). However, it is crucial to acknowledge that shame and guilt are separate emotions. Shame undermines our self-image and contradicts the desires and objectives of our ego. High levels of shame have been linked to negative psychological well-being and functioning. Disorders such as eating disorders, sexual disorders, and even narcissism can be understood as manifestations of shame. On the other hand, guilt aligns with our self-image and is consistent with the needs and goals of our ego. Unless it festers, guilt is either unrelated or inversely correlated with poor psychological functioning.

Sources of Shame and Guilt

Various factors can contribute to different forms of shame and guilt, ranging from temporary triggers to early life experiences, such as growing up in an abusive environment. However, shame and guilt can make themselves known to us in several additional ways, including:

- Facing rejection or the deterioration of relationships

- Mental health disorders involving self-criticism or judgment, such as social anxiety disorder

- Disappointing oneself or experiencing failure

- Struggling to meet excessively high self-imposed standards

- Being subjected to bullying or mistreatment

- Fearing the exposure of flaws or perceived inadequacies

It's worth emphasizing that infants instinctively experience shame, even without explicit learning. In this sense, the initial shame response is a standard and innate part of human development. However, as many of us can attest, when this response becomes excessively intense, it can pose challenges and become problematic.

Developing Forgiveness Techniques for Self and Others

Taking action to address the wrongdoing that led to feelings of shame or guilt is the best way to alleviate these emotions. This may involve apologizing, repairing the damage caused, or making amends. However, self-forgiveness is often necessary to reduce lingering guilt and shame, primarily when forgiveness from others is not obtained. While individuals prone to guilt are more likely to self-forgive, shame-prone individuals may struggle with self-forgiveness.

How to Forgive Yourself

Forgiving yourself can be challenging, but essential for personal growth and healing. When we carry the weight of self-blame and guilt, it hinders our ability to move forward and embrace self-compassion. Fortunately, effective techniques can support the journey of self-forgiveness, allowing us to release the burden of past mistakes and embrace a brighter future.

Self-Reflection

Take time to reflect on the situation and your role in it. Acknowledge your mistakes, shortcomings, and the consequences of your actions. Understand that everyone makes mistakes and that it's part of being human.

Acceptance of Imperfections

Recognize that nobody is perfect, including yourself. Embrace your flaws and imperfections as a natural part of your journey. Remember that making mistakes doesn't define your worth as a person.

Practice Self-Compassion

Treat yourself with kindness, understanding, and forgiveness. Offer yourself the same compassion and empathy that you would to a close friend who made a mistake. Remind yourself that you deserve forgiveness and the opportunity to learn and grow.

Learn From the Experience

Embrace the mistake or wrongdoing as a valuable opportunity for growth and personal development. Engage in introspection to extract the lessons learned and consider how you can steer clear of similar missteps in the future.

Make Amends if Possible

If your actions have harmed others, consider making amends or apologizing. Taking responsibility and expressing genuine remorse can help in the forgiveness process. However, remember that forgiveness is not solely dependent on the response or forgiveness from others.

Release Self-Judgment

Let go of self-blame and self-judgment. Understand that dwelling on guilt and shame serves no purpose and only obstructs your ability to move forward. Remind yourself that you deserve to be forgiven and to experience self-acceptance.

Challenge Negative Self-Talk

Notice and challenge any opposing thoughts or self-talk that may perpetuate guilt or self-condemnation. Replace them with positive and affirming statements that promote self-forgiveness and self-love.

Practice Self-Care

Engage in activities that nourish your well-being and promote self-healing. This can include practicing self-care routines, engaging in hobbies you enjoy, spending time in nature, or seeking professional support through therapy or counseling.

Focus on the Present and Future

Redirect your energy and focus toward the present moment and the future. Set goals, envision positive changes, and commit to personal growth. Allow yourself the opportunity to create a better version of yourself moving forward.

How to Forgive Others

Forgiving others is a transformative act of compassion and liberation. Holding onto grudges and resentment can weigh heavily on our hearts and hinder our personal growth. However, by cultivating forgiveness, we release the burden of anger and pain and create space for healing and restoring relationships. Forgiving others is a powerful journey that requires understanding, empathy, and a willingness to let go of the past. Here are a few techniques I've had to teach myself over the years to forgive those who have profoundly hurt me in the past:

Practice Empathy

Put yourself in the other person's shoes and try to see things from their perspective. Consider factors such as their background, experiences, and personal struggles that may have influenced their behavior.

Understand the Situation

Seek to understand the circumstances and perspectives of the person who hurt you. Try to empathize with their motivations and reasons for their actions.

Express Your Emotions

Allow yourself to acknowledge and express your emotions related to the hurt or betrayal. This can involve talking to a supportive friend or family member, journaling, or seeking therapy.

Let Go of Resentment

Holding onto resentment only prolongs your pain. Choose to release negative feelings and resentment towards the person who hurt you. This doesn't mean forgetting what happened or condoning their actions but freeing yourself from the emotional burden.

Set Boundaries

Establish clear boundaries and communicate them to the person who hurt you. This can help protect yourself from future harm and rebuild trust gradually.

Practice Self-Care

Focus on activities that will benefit your physical and emotional health and help you heal. Look after yourself, and remember to be kind to yourself when working on forgiving others.

Seek Support

Reach out to a therapist, support group, or trusted confidant who can provide guidance and understanding as you navigate the forgiveness journey. Their perspectives and insights can be valuable in gaining clarity and finding closure.

Consider Forgiveness as a Choice

Ultimately, forgiveness is a personal decision. It's not about condoning or forgetting the hurtful actions, but choosing to release the negative emotions and move forward with your life.

Writing Exercises for Releasing Shame and Guilt

Over the years, I've learned that engaging in writing exercises can be a transformative journey toward letting go of shame and guilt. These exercises provide a safe and reflective space to explore emotions, gain clarity, and cultivate self-compassion. Through words, you can release the weight of past mistakes and begin the healing process.

Expressive Journaling

Set aside time to write freely and openly about your shame and guilt. Write without judgment or censorship, allowing your thoughts and emotions to flow onto the paper. Use this space to explore the underlying reasons behind your feelings, reflect on past experiences, and express remorse or self-blame. Writing can provide a cathartic release and help you gain a new perspective on these emotions.

Letter Writing

Write a letter to yourself or the person you feel you have wronged or who has wronged you. Pour out your emotions, expressing your regrets, apologies, and any insights you have gained. This exercise allows you to externalize your feelings and release them onto the paper. You can keep the letter to yourself as a personal practice, or consider sharing it with the intended recipient if it feels appropriate and safe.

Self-Compassion Writing

Focus on cultivating self-compassion through writing. Begin by acknowledging and accepting your imperfections and mistakes. Write compassionate and understanding statements to yourself, emphasizing that mistakes are part of being human. Counter self-judgment with self-compassionate responses, offering forgiveness and kindness to yourself. Affirm your worthiness and remind yourself that you deserve to let go of shame and guilt.

Reframing Exercise

Engage in a reframing exercise by challenging negative self-perceptions associated with shame and guilt. Write down your negative beliefs about yourself and the situations that trigger shame and guilt. Then, write an alternative, more compassionate, and realistic perspective for each belief. Reframe your self-talk by consciously replacing self-blame with self-acceptance and self-forgiveness.

Gratitude Journaling

Practice gratitude journaling to shift your focus from shame and guilt toward positive aspects of your life. Make it a daily habit to jot down three things you're thankful for, no matter how small they may seem. By cultivating a sense of gratitude, you can counterbalance the weight of negative emotions and remind yourself of the good within and around you.

Incorporating Mindfulness-Based Stress Reduction Techniques for Managing Shame and Guilt

Mindfulness-Based Stress Reduction (MBSR) is a program developed by Jon Kabat-Zinn in the 70s to support individuals facing challenges, including physical and mental health issues. While initially designed for hospital patients, MBSR has proven beneficial for diverse populations, transcending backgrounds and circumstances. Its effectiveness extends to people from all walks of life, making it a valuable resource in promoting well-being and resilience.

When incorporated alongside existing medical and psychological interventions, the integration of Mindfulness-Based Stress Reduction has demonstrated its capacity to enhance treatment outcomes across a wide range of conditions and challenges, including:

- sleep problems

- anxiety and panic attacks

- chronic illness

- gastrointestinal distress

- work, family, and financial stress

- cancer

- depression

- heart disease

- fibromyalgia

- skin disorders

- headaches

- high blood pressure

- eating disorders

- fatigue

- post-traumatic stress disorder

- asthma

- pain

- grief (Ackerman, 2017a).

To this list, I would like to add that MBSR has also done wonders for my patients in letting go of shame and guilt. It aids them in cultivating self-compassion and developing a healthier relationship with their emotions. The MBSR techniques that have shown the most promising results include mindful awareness, loving-kindness meditation, RAIN, body scan, and cultivating self-compassion.

Mindful Awareness

Practice bringing non-judgmental awareness to your thoughts, feelings, and bodily sensations related to shame and guilt. Observe them with curiosity and without trying to change or suppress them. This awareness helps you recognize the presence of shame and guilt without getting overwhelmed by them.

Loving-Kindness Meditation

Engage in loving-kindness meditation, directing human and loving thoughts towards yourself and others. This practice helps soften self-judgment and foster self-acceptance, while promoting forgiveness and empathy toward others.

RAIN Technique

RAIN stands for Recognize, Accept, Investigate, and Nurture. When shame or guilt arises, first recognize and acknowledge their presence. Accept the emotions as part of your experience without judgment. Investigate the underlying thoughts, beliefs, and triggers associated with shame and guilt. Finally, nurture yourself with self-compassion and kindness, offering understanding and support.

Body Scan

Perform a body scan meditation, systematically bringing your attention to different body parts. Notice any tension, discomfort, or sensations associated with shame or guilt. This practice helps you develop a non-judgmental relationship with your body and fosters a sense of groundedness and presence.

Cultivating Self-Compassion

Engage in self-compassion exercises, such as writing a self-compassionate letter to yourself or repeating self-compassionate phrases. Treat yourself with the same kindness, understanding, and support you would offer to a loved one facing similar challenges.

Incorporating Rational Emotive Behavior Therapy (REBT) Techniques for Assertiveness Training

Next, we will dive into a cognitive behavioral therapy (CBT) method created by psychologist Albert Ellis called the Rational Emotive Behavior Therapy (REBT). This therapeutic approach is designed to actively assist people in addressing irrational beliefs and developing skills to effectively handle their emotions, thoughts, and behaviors more rationally.

Clinging to irrational beliefs about ourselves or the world can lead to various challenges and difficulties. REBT aims to enable us to identify and modify these beliefs and negative thinking patterns, ultimately helping us to overcome psychological issues and alleviate mental distress. By working on reframing our perspectives and adopting more rational and constructive thoughts, we can achieve improved emotional well-being and a healthier approach to life's challenges.

REBT offers various techniques for assertiveness training to help people develop practical communication skills and confidently express their needs and boundaries. Here are some REBT techniques commonly used in assertiveness training:

ABC Model

The ABC model is a foundational component of REBT. It helps people identify the activating event (A), their beliefs and interpretations about the event (B), and the emotional and behavioral consequences (C) that result from those beliefs. By challenging and restructuring irrational beliefs, you can develop more assertive responses. Here's how you can apply this model:

- Identify an activating event that triggered an emotional response or led to passive or aggressive behavior.

- Write down your beliefs and thoughts about the event.

- Analyze and challenge your irrational beliefs by asking yourself questions like: "What evidence supports or contradicts this belief?", "What are the alternative interpretations?", "Is this belief helpful or constructive?"

- Restructure your beliefs by replacing irrational thoughts with more rational and realistic ones.

- Reflect on how changing your beliefs could lead to more assertive responses in similar situations.

Disputing Irrational Beliefs

REBT encourages individuals to identify and dispute irrational beliefs that hinder assertiveness. This involves questioning the validity and usefulness of irrational thoughts and replacing them with more rational and constructive beliefs. Here's how to do it:

- Write down one of your irrational beliefs about assertiveness, such as "If I assert myself, people will dislike me."

- Examine the evidence that supports this belief and the evidence that contradicts it.

- Generate rational counterstatements that challenge the irrational belief, such as "Asserting myself allows me to express my needs and values, and healthy relationships respect assertiveness."

- Repeat the rational counterstatements to yourself regularly, replacing the irrational belief with a more rational perspective.

Role-Playing

Role-playing exercises provide a safe environment to practice assertive behaviors and responses. Individuals can simulate challenging situations and actively work on expressing their needs, setting boundaries, and responding assertively. Here's an exercise to get you started:

- Identify a specific assertiveness scenario you find challenging, such as asking for a raise or setting boundaries with a friend.

- Enlist the help of a trusted friend or therapist to role-play the scenario.

- Practice expressing your needs, setting boundaries, and responding assertively in the role-play scenario.

- Receive feedback from your partner and make adjustments as necessary.

- Repeat the role-play exercise multiple times to enhance your assertiveness and confidence.

Self-Assertion Training

This technique involves teaching individuals specific skills and strategies for assertive communication. It may include techniques such as "I-statements" (expressing feelings and needs using "I feel" or "I want"), active listening, assertive body language, and effective negotiation. Here's how you can begin your self-assertion training:

- Choose a specific situation where you want to practice assertiveness, such as expressing a disagreement at work.

- Write down an "I-statement" that clearly communicates your thoughts, feelings, and needs relating to the situation.

- Practice delivering the "I-statement" in front of a mirror, focusing on using assertive body language and tone of voice.

- Visualize the scenario, imagining yourself confidently expressing your needs using the "I-statement."

- Role-play the situation with a supportive friend or therapist, receiving feedback and refining your assertive communication skills.

Rational Self-Talk

REBT emphasizes the importance of cultivating rational and empowering self-talk. I've had substantial success developing assertiveness by teaching myself to identify negative self-statements and replace them with positive, self-affirming thoughts supporting assertiveness and self-confidence. The following exercise is one I use frequently:

- Identify a situation where you tend to engage in negative self-talk or self-doubt related to assertiveness.

- Write down your negative self-statements, such as "I'm not good at asserting myself."

- Challenge these negative statements by questioning their validity and replacing them with positive and empowering self-talk, such as "I have the right to express myself assertively, and I am capable of doing so."

- Repeat the positive self-talk statements regularly, particularly before entering assertiveness situations, to reinforce a more confident and assertive mindset.

Gradual Exposure

This technique involves gradually exposing individuals to increasingly challenging assertiveness situations. Starting with less intimidating scenarios and progressively working up to more difficult ones can help you build confidence and develop assertive behaviors over time. Here's how you can gradually expose yourself to these types of scenarios:

- Create a list of assertiveness scenarios ranked from least challenging to most challenging.

- Start by practicing assertiveness in the least intimidating scenario, such as asking a friend for a small favor.

- Once you feel comfortable, gradually progress to more challenging situations, such as expressing a differing opinion in a group setting or negotiating a compromise.

- Reflect on each experience, noting your successes and areas for improvement, and use them as learning opportunities to build your assertiveness skills.

Homework Assignments

I like to assign homework tasks related to assertiveness to my patients, which helps them practice and apply assertive techniques in real-life situations. It may involve journaling assertive interactions, reflecting on challenges and successes, or setting assertiveness goals for oneself. You can also assign these tasks to yourself, including:

- Keeping a journal of assertive interactions throughout the week.

- Writing down instances where you successfully expressed your needs assertively and the positive outcomes that resulted.

- Reflect on any challenges or setbacks you faced and explore strategies for improvement.

- Setting assertiveness goals for yourself, such as practicing assertiveness in a specific situation or increasing the frequency of assertive communication.

- Regularly review your journal and track your progress to boost motivation and self-awareness

Understanding the Process of Integration

Integration is a dynamic process that involves merging distinct groups or entities into a cohesive whole. For example, integrating various software systems or applications in the technology field allows for seamless data sharing and communication between different platforms. This integration enhances efficiency, productivity, and user experience by eliminating the need for manual data transfer and enabling interoperability.

In personal development, however, integration can be understood as the harmonious blending of different aspects of an individual's identity or personality. For instance, someone undergoing self-reflection and personal growth may strive to integrate their values, beliefs, and behaviors, leading to a more authentic and congruent sense of self. Overall, integration manifests in various domains of life, promoting inclusivity, efficiency, growth, and synergy by bringing together diverse elements into a unified and functional whole.

Creating a Self-Care Plan for Ongoing Healing

Integration and creating a self-care plan go hand-in-hand because both involve recognizing and embracing the various aspects of oneself, bringing together separate parts, and fostering a sense of wholeness and balance. Integrating different aspects of our lives and addressing our physical, emotional, and mental well-being through self-care can create a solid foundation for personal growth, healing, and well-being.

Now, let's explore some practical self-care techniques to support us in this journey toward holistic well-being. These techniques aim to nourish our mind, body, and spirit and empower us to cultivate self-awareness, resilience, and inner strength.

Don't make the same mistake as I did on my healing journey by viewing self-care as a luxury. On the contrary, it's a vital component of our healing process. We can foster greater balance, peace, and fulfillment by dedicating time and attention to ourselves.

Assess Your Needs

Begin by assessing your physical, emotional, and mental well-being. Identify areas in your life that require healing and self-care. This could include managing stress, addressing emotional trauma, improving sleep patterns, nurturing relationships, and maintaining a healthy lifestyle.

Set Realistic Goals

Establish achievable goals that align with your healing journey. Break them down into smaller, manageable steps to prevent becoming overwhelmed. For example, if you're focusing on emotional healing, a goal might be to practice self-compassion and positive affirmations daily.

Identify Self-Care Activities

Explore various self-care practices that resonate with you. These can be activities that promote relaxation, self-reflection, creativity, or physical well-being. Examples include meditation, journaling, engaging in hobbies, exercise, spending time in nature, or seeking therapy.

Establish a Routine

Create a consistent self-care routine that integrates these activities into your daily or weekly schedule. Make self-care a priority and allocate dedicated time for it. Consider using reminders or setting specific time blocks to ensure regular self-care practice.

Seek Support

If you need assistance, don't hesitate to contact your support system or seek guidance from a professional. This can include friends, family, support groups, or therapists who can provide advice, understanding, and validation during your healing journey.

Practice Self-Compassion

Be gentle with yourself and practice self-compassion throughout the healing process. Acknowledge that healing takes time and effort. Embrace setbacks as opportunities for growth and learning, and celebrate the small victories.

Adjust and Adapt

Continuously reassess your self-care plan and make adjustments as needed. Your needs and priorities may change as you evolve and progress in your healing journey. Stay open to new self-care strategies and be willing to adapt your plan accordingly.

Incorporating a self-care plan for ongoing healing into your life is a transformative journey toward self-nurturing and personal growth. By regularly assessing your needs, setting realistic goals, and engaging in activities that replenish your well-being, you create a solid foundation for ongoing healing.

Guided Meditation for Integrating the Inner Child

To further guide you on using integration for healing, I have recorded two more guided meditations, which you can access via the QR code below.

These guided meditations are designed to support your inner growth, allowing you to connect with your inner self and harness the power of your breath to facilitate integration and healing. Prepare yourself for a calming and rejuvenating experience as you embark on this self-care practice.

Scan Me

Grounding Meditation for Integration

1. To start, get into a comfortable seated position with a straight spine and relaxed body. Close your eyes and take a deep breath, filling your lungs and slowly exhaling. As you breathe deeply, focus on your body and feel the weight of it being supported by the surface you're sitting on.

2. Now, shift your attention to your feet. Visualize roots growing from the soles of your feet, extending deep into the Earth. With each breath, imagine these roots becoming more substantial and deeply rooted. Feel the stability and grounding energy flowing from the Earth, grounding you in the present moment.

3. Take a moment to focus on your breathing. As you inhale, visualize yourself taking in positive, healing energy. And as you exhale, release any stored tension or negative energy. With each breath, connect more deeply with yourself and the present moment.

4. Now, envision a gentle light surrounding your body. This light represents the integration of all aspects of yourself, your experiences, and your emotions. As you continue to breathe, allow

this light to expand and fill your entire being. Feel a sense of harmony and wholeness as all parts of you come together in perfect unity.

5. Stay in this state of integration for a few moments, bathing in the healing light and the sense of oneness. Whenever you're ready, slowly bring your awareness back to your surroundings, gently open your eyes, and carry the energy of integration throughout your day.

Scan Me

Loving-Kindness Meditation for Integration

1. To begin, find a quiet place and close your eyes. Take several deep breaths and release any tension you may be feeling. Once you feel calm and relaxed, think of someone important to you supporting your growth and recovery. This person could be a family member, a close friend, or a mentor.

2. Visualize this person standing in front of you, radiating love and compassion. Feel their presence and the warmth of their unconditional support. As you connect with this person's energy, silently repeat the following phrases.

3. "May you experience true happiness. May you enjoy optimal health. May you find safety and security. May your life be filled with ease and tranquility."

4. Allow these phrases to resonate within you as you genuinely wish this person love, happiness, and well-being. Feel the energy of love expanding within your heart, embracing the interconnectedness between you and this individual.

5. Now, gradually shift your focus to yourself. Recognize that you, too, deserve love, happiness, and well-being. Silently repeat the exact phrases, directing them towards yourself.

6. "May I experience true happiness. May I enjoy optimal health. May I find safety and security. May my life be filled with ease and tranquility."

7. Feel the warmth of these words filling your entire being, nurturing your self-acceptance and self-compassion. Embrace the truth that integration begins with self-love and acceptance.

Spend a few extra minutes soaking up the positive, loving energy and let it seep into every part of your body. When you're ready, bring your attention back to the present moment and continue your day, carrying the energy of love and integration.

Incorporating Positive Psychology Techniques for Maintaining Inner Child Healing

By incorporating the practice of positive psychology techniques into your daily life, you can provide ongoing support, nurture, and healing to your inner child, fostering a deep sense of self-compassion and inner harmony. Through the lens of positive psychology, these techniques empower you to maintain a strong connection with your inner child, ensuring their continued healing and integration into your present life. Remember to try and practice the following below:

Self-Compassion

Cultivate self-compassion by treating yourself with kindness, understanding, and acceptance. Practice self-care, self-acceptance, and self-forgiveness to support and nurture your inner child.

Inner Child Check-Ins

Regularly check in with your inner child through mindfulness or meditation practices. Set aside moments of quiet reflection to connect with your inner child, listen to their needs, and provide reassurance and love.

Inner Child Journaling

Continue journaling to explore and understand your inner child's needs, desires, and emotions. Use your journal to express gratitude, reflect on progress, and identify areas requiring further healing or attention.

Creative Expression

Engage in creative activities that allow self-expression and exploration of your inner child. This could include art, music, dance, writing, or any other creative outlet that resonates with you. Allow your inner child to express themselves freely through these creative endeavors.

Inner Child Rituals

Create rituals or habits that cater to the needs of your inner child. This may mean doing activities that bring joy, comfort, or playfulness to your inner child, like walking in nature, playing games, or pursuing hobbies and interests that make you happy.

Inner Child Affirmations and Mantras

Continue using affirmations and positive self-talk to reinforce healing messages and nurture your inner child. Affirmations can remind you of your worthiness, resilience, and capacity for growth. Repeat affirmations or mantras regularly to reinforce positive beliefs and thoughts.

Inner Child Support Network

Surround yourself with understanding and supportive people who can encourage, empathize, and validate your inner child's healing journey. Seek therapists, support groups, or like-minded individuals who can offer guidance and a safe space for sharing experiences.

By practicing self-compassion, engaging in inner child check-ins, expressing yourself creatively, and cultivating a supportive network, you create a nurturing environment for your inner child to thrive. These techniques provide the foundation for maintaining the healing and growth that has begun, allowing you to embrace your authentic self and live a life filled with joy, resilience, and self-acceptance. May your ongoing journey of inner child healing be a source of empowerment and transformation, enriching every aspect of your life

'Equip yourself
with the tools
of DBT, and
empower
yourself to
navigate life's
challenges with
resilience.'

Marsha Linehan

——

CHAPTER 10

——

Dialectical Behavioral Therapy (DBT)

In this final chapter, we will dive further into Dialectical Behavioral Therapy (DBT) to help you understand how it can help you on this journey and how to even practice it on a daily basis. DBT is a type of cognitive-behavioral therapy that focuses on helping people change negative thinking patterns and behaviors. This technique is important because it teaches skills that can help you improve your mental health in a manageable and positive way.

DBT was originally created to treat borderline personality disorder (BPD), but has proven effective in treating a variety of mental health conditions, such as depression, anxiety, and eating disorders (Schimelpfening, 2021).

DBT skills are divided into four major categories:

- mindfulness
- distress tolerance
- emotion regulation
- interpersonal effectiveness

DBT is important as it can help you to:

- identify and label emotions
- express emotions healthily
- tolerate difficult emotions
- regulate emotions
- set boundaries in relationships
- communicate effectively

Although this type of therapy was originally developed to treat certain mental health disorders, it can effectively help anyone who would like to improve their emotion regulation and communication techniques. DBT is especially helpful for people who struggle with emotions, communication, or relationships, regardless of the state of their mental health.

DBT usually consists of weekly individual therapy sessions and group skills training sessions. Skills training sessions are typically two to three hours long, and are held once a week. In total, it usually takes about six months to a year to complete.

Five years into my practice, I met an incredibly successful young woman, Jan. Jan was younger than me, in her mid-twenties, and had her own company that she built from the ground up in two years. Within the first year, she was already making a profit and the following year, she pocketed half a million dollars. She was engaged to an equally successful man and together they had a five-year plan that included a family, more businesses, and more wealth.

Within the following year, they planned to marry and enjoy their honeymoon. Year two would be a home purchase and the next three years would be spent working on their family and their home. Overall, Jan was beautiful, smart, and had an enviable life. But despite all of her success, Jan was not happy. In fact, she was really struggling.

She came to see me because she was desperate. She had been to therapy before in college and tried medication, but nothing seemed to help. When I asked her what was going on, she told me she just couldn't seem to stop herself from self-deprecating behaviors. No matter how much she wanted to, or how bad the consequences were, she just couldn't stop thinking negatively, she was worrying excessively, and when it got to be too much, she often turned to alcohol or drugs to offset the mental anguish within.

I asked her to tell me more about these behaviors and she said that they provided her with short-term relief from the pain she was feeling inside, but these behaviors were actually making her life worse. They were costing her money, ruining relationships, and causing her immense amounts of shame and guilt. She needed a new method to deal with her emotions and that's when I suggested DBT.

DBT focuses on helping people change negative thinking and behaviors by teaching them new skills. The word "dialectical" means "the art of finding the middle ground" (Rosie, 2020). In other words, it's about learning to see both sides of a situation and finding a balance between them.

This therapy technique can be difficult to understand and apply at first, but Jan found it helpful to think of it as a set of skills that she could learn in order to deal with her emotions in a more productive way. Each month, we would focus on a unique skill and Jan would practice using it in her everyday life. Some skills were a little challenging for Jan, such as learning how to be more mindful, but with time and practice, she saw results.

Within a few months, Jan was feeling better than she had in years. She was still successful at work and in her relationship, but she could also cope with her emotions healthily. Her fiancé noticed an improvement as well and was supportive of her continued progress, which strengthened their relationship. DBT had given her the tools she needed to manage her emotions and create a life that was balanced and fulfilling. This therapy technique has changed Jan's life for the better and I am proud to say that she is now one of my success stories.

If you have been struggling with negative thinking or self-destructive behaviors, this treatment may help you too. In this chapter, you will learn about:

- dialectical behavior therapy and how it was developed
- how this approach works and what happens in therapy
- the benefits and how it can help you

For your last step in this journey, we will learn more about this type of therapy and how it can change your life for the better.

What Exactly Is Dialectical Behavior Therapy?

DBT is a combination of cognitive-behavioral therapy and mindfulness techniques. The cognitive-behavioral part will help you learn to identify and change the thoughts or behaviors that are keeping you stuck in ruts. The mindfulness approach will teach you how to be present in the moment and accept yourself just as you are so you can learn to appreciate life more.

This form of talk therapy is an evidence-based approach, with success rates higher than most treatments out there today for eating disorders, depression, anxiety, and other mental health issues. Like with Jan, the overall goal is to help you develop skills to deal with intense emotions, impulsive behaviors, and self-destructive thoughts. These thoughts are normal, but they can be harmful if we don't know how to deal with them.

History of DBT

DBT was developed in the 1980s by Marsha Linehan, a professor of psychology at the University of Washington. Linehan was originally trained in behavioral therapy, but she found it was not effective in treating borderline personality disorder. She combined Eastern philosophies, such as Buddhism, and Western philosophies, to create this method, which makes it more effective than either on its own!

The DBT Process

This approach is based on the principle that you are capable of change and, by teaching you new, yet practical skills, you can transform your behaviors, thoughts, and emotions. Remember, after a few months Jan noticed a tremendous improvement in her ability to communicate and handle challenges. The tools she learned allowed her to focus on the four critical areas in DBT: mindfulness practice, interpersonal effectiveness training, distress tolerance, and emotion regulation.

These techniques will help you learn how to balance needs and wants in relationships with others and understand what makes you happy or sad without judging those emotions themselves. This also involves learning how to communicate in a way that allows others to understand your wants and needs. From there, you can work on managing your own emotions better through mindful techniques. For example, you might write down lists when you're angry so it doesn't boil over into something more harmful. Lastly, you will learn how to be more effective in crisis situations so that you don't feel as if you're losing control.

This approach acknowledges that we all have different sides to our personality, and it's important for people like you who are struggling to find a balance between these two poles so you can live in relative calm. For example, you may possess an impulsive side, which often gets expressed through rash decisions or actions while, at other times, doing things with thoughtful care.

However, this doesn't mean one was better than another, but either could get lost if they're not balanced against each other properly. The unbalance can lead you down an unhealthy path towards disaster! However, there's hope, though, thanks again to DBT—this time through mindfulness practices rather than traditional psychotherapy exercises—you can find your own happy medium where both elements work together nicely without vying over control of them all the time.

What DBT Is Not

The goal of this technique is not to tell you what your next move should be, but rather empower you with the tools and knowledge necessary for self-harmony to help you improve yourself by understanding your emotional reactions so you can make healthier decisions in the future. It's not the cure-all for mental health disorders, but it can help you manage them and live a happier life with more balance in mind!

Who Should Try This Approach?

This innovative form of therapy has been effective in treating many mental health disorders, but can help anyone in many aspects of their lives. If you are struggling with any mental health concerns and want an easier way out, then DBT may ease some challenges by teaching coping skills. Even if this isn't something affecting your life currently, dialectics will help you cultivate healthier living habits which include being more mindful and happier.

This approach focuses on changing your thoughts and behaviors, while promoting mindfulness. It can help you learn to accept yourself, while also teaching how you process your thoughts and feelings within yourself with the help of dialectics (the middle way). Then you can go about changing your beliefs or behaviors that are causing you distress. DBT also has many resources for reducing stress or enhancing self-awareness, so it may be right if you struggle with these issues currently.

What Happens in Dialectical Behavior Therapy?

In therapy, you would learn how to change the negative patterns you indulge in by using long-lasting techniques. You can work one on one with a therapist in individual sessions to learn how it works. Then practice these skills outside of therapy when possible.

You can also learn these techniques during group practices where other people are learning the same thing from instructors too—this way you can help each other get better while receiving support. The number of sessions you attend will depend on your individual needs.

What Benefits Can I Receive?

This treatment focuses on fighting against negative thoughts and rewarding good ones, which gives you more control over your emotions. You can feel like you have more power over your life by learning how you can handle difficult situations when they arise in everyday life (like setting boundaries). With DBT, there's no need to feel like a victim anymore because this approach aims at empowering you so you don't give up on yourself but take control instead

DBT focuses on four areas: mindfulness, interpersonal effectiveness, emotion regulation, and distress tolerance.

Mindfulness

Mindfulness is the practice of being present in the moment, where you become aware of your thoughts and feelings without judgment. It's helpful to think of this technique as a muscle you can strengthen with practice. Many activities are available that you can perform to strengthen this muscle, including meditation, yoga, and deep breathing exercises.

For instance, mindful eating is a great way to promote mindfulness as it focuses entirely on what you're putting into your body. The act of actually experiencing the taste, smell, or touch can be very empowering because, when we focus too much attention, only one thought comes up: *I'm hungry*. It may sound silly but this really opens our minds back up again. Instead of focusing on the negative ions caused by all these other unimportant factors such as social status at work, etc., you can focus on the task at hand which is eating.

These methods help us learn more about self-awareness while also allowing space between what feels good (stimuli) or bad (distress). Mindfulness can also help you to:

- be more present in your life
- accept yourself and others
- make better decisions
- communicate more effectively
- handle difficult emotions

Interpersonal Effectiveness

Interpersonal effectiveness can help you improve the quality of relationships in your life. These interpersonal effectiveness skills will provide a comforting way for you to set boundaries and assert yourself in relationships, whether they are personal or professional ones! Yelling at your partner is unnecessary when you have tailored techniques which allows you to communicate better at raising your voice or being aggressive. Examples of these techniques include:

- active listening
- assertive communication

- negotiation
- conflict resolution

Emotion Regulation

The third principle is to learn emotion regulation skills. Emotionally intelligent people manage their emotions and reduce stress, which helps them be more productive both personally and professionally with clients or colleagues alike! Examples of these techniques include:

- identifying and labeling emotions
- recognizing early warning signs of distress
- developing a plan to cope with difficult emotions
- relaxation and self-soothing techniques

Distress Tolerance

Distress tolerance skills can help you understand your tolerated level of anger (with oneself and others) while having healthier coping strategies. For instance, you might learn problem solving skills to combat worrying about what might go wrong. Overall, these skills allow you to stand proud of who we are despite any setbacks.

The DBT skills teach a kind and effective way to deal with difficult situations, emotions, or relationships. These techniques will assist you during your personal life, but if used professionally, they can make an excellent difference too. The key component about these exercises is that they should be done gradually—you can't just suddenly start applying them when you're already stressed out! Examples of these techniques include:

- dialectical reasoning
- distraction
- self-soothing
- acceptance

The Five Key Principles

DBT is an approach to treatment that focuses on helping people to accept and change their behaviors. The goal of this technique is not to control or suppress emotions, but to help you understand them so you can work through them. These key principles guide therapists in helping their patients to understand the following:

- dialectics
- change is inevitable
- acceptance and change are not mutually exclusive
- all behavior has a purpose
- progress, not perfection

Human beings are constantly changing creatures. The first principle, dialectics, is the idea that everything changes and that there are two sides to every story. This helps you to understand how others may see things differently than you do. The principle also validates a patients' feelings during therapy sessions. Feeling like you're the only one who truly knows what is going on in your life at any given time because of changes occurring around you regularly is common.

The second principle is that change is inevitable. This means you can't prevent or stop all the surrounding differences—but this also makes them part of what we call *life*. That change is a natural part of life that can be challenging to accept, but it's important for people who experience unexpected events in their lives or relationships. Changes may come about due either situationally (elderly parents) and/or relationally (divorce). Understanding how these factors affect you, then, allows you to take steps towards managing any emotions you might experience.

This third principle is the idea that people can accept their current situation while also working towards change. It helps you understand you may need to embrace some aspects of yourself before being able to make any noticeable changes in your life or behaviors. For example, if you're trying to lose weight, you may need to come to terms with your specific body type and how it processes food before making any serious dietary changes. This often leads you to a path where you can accept your current situation and then work toward changing whatever needs fixing from there.

The fourth principle is that all behavior has a purpose. Even if the behavior itself is unhealthy, your behaviors are connected to an extent and are necessary. Your behaviors are driven by desire without randomness and when you can understand this, then everything starts to make sense. This means that your actions have a reason behind them. You may not be aware of what's motivating you, but it could very well come from an authentic place within yourself. Even if it's something as simple as wanting attention or approval, you still need to check in with yourself before acting on these desires. Otherwise, there might be side effects later when those needs aren't being met anymore.

This ultimate principle is about the importance of progress over perfection. This means being more accommodating to yourself and others by understanding that you will make mistakes. It also helps therapists focus on what's important rather than trying to be perfect all the time. Think like an artist who knows their brushstrokes aren't always perfect but focuses more so on getting good at painting strokes instead. The same idea here, taking baby steps might seem like a slower process, but it sets you up for success in the long-run.

These five key principles guide therapists in helping others, like you, to change. It creates a basis for therapists to provide better care for their patients and help them achieve their goals.

Four Functions of Therapy and How a Therapist Can Help You

Four principal functions form DBT: motivating individuals, teaching skills, generalizing skills to natural environments, and structuring the treatment environment.

Motivating individuals: People struggling with mental health issues often have difficulty motivating themselves to seek treatment and participate in therapy. This is where the DBT approach comes into play: by using several techniques such as providing support, structure (throughout the week), positive reinforcement.

for taking part in therapy sessions, it's possible that people will be more likely than ever before to be motivated enough to attend and also complete their care plan!

Teaching skills: This type of counseling teaches people skills to cope with difficult emotions, manage stress, and improve their relationships. It's taught through individual, group, or self-help techniques like homework assignments so therapists can give feedback on how you're doing throughout your sessions.

Generalizing skills to natural environments: This therapy technique helps clients generalize the skills they learn in therapy in their everyday lives. This is accomplished by providing support and structure outside of treatment, using real-life examples during sessions (such as family members), and practicing these new behaviors everyday so it becomes second nature for you!

Structuring the treatment environment: DBT skills has various techniques to structure the treatment environment in a way that is supportive and helpful for clients, such as providing support or framework during sessions. One technique used by this approach includes having therapists partake themselves so you could experience firsthand what it feels like on both sides of an issue—the person who holds negative attitudes towards their problem while also being part physician helping patients deal with these problems more effectively through therapy!

Some people may be genetically predisposed to having mood disorders, but the good news is that there's something you can do about it! DBT can assist you with learning skills to cope with difficult situations in life more constructively than before. By learning new techniques on how to handle emotions differently without resorting back to old habits linked with negative thinking patterns, you can really make all the difference when going through hard times.

'You are the master of your destiny. You can influence, direct, and control your own environment.'

Napoleon Hill

———

CHAPTER 11

Changing Your Mindset

In order for DBT to be successful, it's important that you understand and accept the changes listed below.

- You must be patient with yourself during this journey of self-discovery and growth—it's not an "all or nothing" approach.
- No one is perfect—we all make mistakes. It's part of being human! What counts the most is that you're taking steps towards improving your life and relationships for the better.
- You will have many opportunities for success along the way because there are many techniques you can choose from when it comes down to deciding what kind(s) of coping methods would work best in any situation.
- The goal isn't about *fixing,* but finding new coping methods for life challenges which will lead to a more fulfilling, happier life in general.

- At times, often during very stressful ones, you may feel stuck. Don't worry though—you'll be learning something new to combat those struggles.
- This approach requires an open mind even when evidence seems repugnant or counterintuitive. An open mind allows you to bounce back from challenging moments without getting stuck in self-hate—the goal is to learn how to make challenges more easy to manage, not worse.
- Self-compassion also allows you to be more honest with yourself.
    - You can admit your mistakes and shortcomings without beating yourself up. You can learn from your failures instead of letting them define you. Then you can approach your life with a sense of curiosity and wonder, rather than judgment and criticism.
- Dialectics focuses on the idea that conflict must have resolutions with both sides. This helps you see a situation from different perspectives so you are more likely to hear what others may believe or how they feel about an issue at hand without getting caught up in your own emotions along the way.

Learning these skills takes time, but eventually your brain waves will change and create new neural pathways for healthier thinking patterns. This can lead you to a calmer, more content state overall. To help you, I have crafted a 7 week programme below that would introduce you to the basics of mindfulness and its importance in this therapy technique. I recommend that you bookmark this page and read it first thing in the morning to practice the techniques for the relevant week.

THE 7 WEEK DBT PROGRAMME-

WEEK 1 - Mindfulness

- Mindfulness is a key component of DBT and refers to the practice of being present in the moment and paying attention to your thoughts, feelings, and surroundings without judgment.
- There are four types of mindfulness: observing, describing, participating, and non-reactivity.
- There are many benefits to being mindful, including reducing stress, anxiety, and depression.
- Mindfulness can be practiced in various ways, such as through meditation, yoga, or walking. It is important to find what works best for you so you don't lose interest and will practice regularly.
- This technique takes time and practice to develop, but it is worth the effort!
- Now that you have read about mindfulness, it's time to put it into practice! Below are some exercises to help you get started.

Action Steps

1. Determine which mindfulness technique you want to work on first: mind, body, breath, or *dhamma*.
2. Find a quiet place to sit or lie down. Close your eyes and take a few deep breaths.
3. Notice your thoughts and emotions without judgment or reactivity.
4. If your mind wanders, simply bring your attention back to your breath.
5. Continue for 5-10 minutes.

Practice this exercise regularly and notice how your relationship with your thoughts and emotions changes

WEEK 2 - Practicing mindfulness skills

- Mindfulness is the act of purposely paying attention to the present moment without reacting or judging them.
- One mind means that everything and everybody is connected. We're all part of the same *dhamma*.
- The act of being mindful includes observing and describing your emotions, thoughts, body, and mind with an open mind and without judging them.
- Mindfulness is an effective way to reduce stress and anxiety. It can also help improve mood, sleep, and overall well-being.

Action Steps

1. Choose one of the mindfulness practices above to focus on: mind, body, thoughts, or emotions.
2. Make a commitment to practice mindfulness for a set period each day.
3. Notice and log the benefits that you experience from practicing mindfulness.
4. Keep a journal to log your experiences with mindfulness. This can be a helpful way to track your progress and see the benefits that you're experiencing. Include feelings, thoughts, situations that occurred during your practice, and anything else that you feel is relevant. Also, include what happened throughout your day. If you settled into a mindful practice with negative thoughts, why?
5. If you struggle with mindfulness, seek a therapist or counselor who can help you. There are many resources available to help you get started with mindfulness and to support you in your journey.

WEEK 3 - Accepting current situation and managing crisis using distress tolerance

- Distress tolerance is a set of skills that can help you deal with challenging situations healthily, which can help you feel more in control of your life.
- You can practice distress tolerance using a variety of methods, such as by volunteering, practicing radical acceptance, improving the moment or situation, or using the acronyms to self-soothe and distract you from turmoil.

Three popular acronyms to help you with distress tolerance are TIPP (Temperature, Intense Exercise, Paced Breathing, Paired Muscle Relaxation), ACCEPTS (Activities, Contribute, Comparison, Emotions, Pushing Away, Thoughts, Sensations), and STOP (Stop! Take a Step Back. Observe. and Proceed Mindfully).

Action Steps

1. For each day of the week, try a different distress tolerance activity. For example, your schedule might look something like this:
   a. Monday: thoughts
   b. Tuesday: sensations
   c. Wednesday: radical acceptance
   d. Thursday: pros and cons lists
   e. Friday: visualization
   f. Saturday: mindfulness
   g. Sunday: self-soothing

Remember that there is no right or wrong way to do this. The important thing is that you're taking the time to focus on distress tolerance and to notice the benefits that you experience.

2. Keep a journal with the benefits that you notice, as well as any drawbacks or anything you feel might apply to the experience.

3. Determine which ones you like the most and are most beneficial to your routine or goals.
   Set aside time every day to perform a distress tolerance activities

WEEK 4 – Identify, name and change your emotions

- Emotions are a normal and essential part of your experience. They provide information about what's going on inside of your mind and bodies and can be helpful in guiding your behavior, but should be regulated properly.
- Big emotions are a normal part of life, but emotions don't equal weakness, only that you're human.
- Some emotion regulation techniques include identifying your emotions, accepting your emotions, labeling your emotions, describing your emotions, expressing your emotions productively, refocusing your attention, and problem solving.
- The benefits of emotion regulation are improved mental and physical health, enhanced well-being, increased life satisfaction, better relationships, and greater work productivity.

Action Steps

1. Identify the signs that convey that you need help to regulate your emotions, such as impulsive decision making, self-harm, or difficulty communicating how you're feeling.
2. Determine which emotions you struggle with the most, such as happiness, sadness, anger, fear, disgust, or surprise.
3. Think about what might trigger these emotions for you, like a certain person, place, or thing.
4. Identify any unhealthy coping mechanisms you use to deal with your emotions like drinking, drugs, self-harm, or impulsive decision making.
5. Develop a plan of action to deal with your emotions healthily with the help of a therapist or other professional.

Start practicing some emotion regulation techniques like problem solving, refocusing your attention, or expressing your emotions healthily.

WEEK 5 - Having more positive emotional experiences with emotion regulation.

- You can manage emotions by speaking kindly and positively to yourself, which can help you feel happier and cope with challenges productively.
- You can use ABC PLEASE to help you manage emotions by accumulating positive experience, building mastery, coping ahead, and treating physical illness.
- You can practice managing emotions by taking the opposite action of what the emotion is telling you to do.

Action Steps

1. If you're feeling an emotion that is intense or overwhelming, try using the STOP skill. STOP stands for stop, take a step back, observe, and proceed mindfully, which helps you assess the situation from a different perspective.

2. Try using positive self-talk to manage your emotions. This means speaking to yourself compassionately. Try saying *I'm a good person* or *I'm trying my hardest.* This type of positive self-talk can help you cope with your emotions or thoughts and develop more confidence.

3. If you're feeling an emotion that makes you uncomfortable, try using the opposite action skill and practice the opposite response. This can help ease emotion's symptoms and prevent you from acting unhealthily.

4. Try using the ABC PLEASE (Accumulating positive emotions, Building mastery, Coping ahead, PLEASE (treating Physical illness, balancing Eating, avoiding substances, balancing Sleep, and getting Exercise) skill to manage your emotions. This is a skill that

can help you take care of yourself in a more holistic way, which can help you manage your emotions more effectively.

WEEK 6 - Communicating more assertively with interpersonal effectiveness.

- It is important to have limits in order to maintain your independence and autonomy.
- There are two types of boundaries: physical and emotional.
- Physical boundaries include your personal space and bodies. Emotional boundaries include your thoughts, feelings, and opinions.
- It is important to communicate assertively in order to maintain healthy relationships.

The THINK (True, Helpful, Inspiring, Necessary, and Kind) acronym is a helpful tool that can help you communicate assertively. For example, is what you are saying True, or is it baseless assumptions? Is what you are saying Helpful? Does it Inspire others? Is what you are saying Necessary? Are the words Kind?

Reflection Questions

- Are you assertive or aggressive? Can you pinpoint the difference between the two using examples from your life?
- How do you think the THINK acronym can help you communicate more assertively and respectfully in your everyday life?
- What do you think are some benefits of communicating assertively? Some consequences of not communicating assertively may include feeling like you can't trust the other person or getting hurt. What are some other possible consequences?

- Think about a time when you could not communicate your needs assertively. What were the circumstances of that event? What resulted from not being assertive?
- Now, think about a time when you could communicate your needs assertively. What were the circumstances of that event? What resulted from being assertive?

  What do you think are some reasons people have trouble communicating assertively? Can you think of any solutions to help overcome these reasons?

WEEK 7 - Clarifying your goals in relationship and maintaining your self respect.

- Self-respect is important in order to have healthy and happy relationships. When you have self-respect, you are more likely to be respected by others.
- You can have self-respect by setting boundaries, communicating your needs, and being truthful.
- The acronym FAST will help you be more effective in having self-respect.
- DEAR MAN can help you be assertive in asking for what you need.
- GIVE can help you learn how to compromise without sacrificing your needs.

Action steps

- Set boundaries in order to protect your time, energy, and resources.
- Communicate your needs assertively using "I" statements.
- Be truthful to yourself and others.
- Use the acronym FAST (Fair, Apologies, Stick to values, and Truthful) to help you be more effective in having self-respect.
- DBT uses the "DEAR MAN" strategy to help you properly communicate with others and make requests. Each letter

represents a different step in the process, which consists of the following: Describe, Express, Assert, Reinforce, Mindfully ask, Appear confident, and Negotiate.

- Practice using the DEAR MAN technique to assertively ask for what you need.
- Learn how to compromise without sacrificing your needs using the GIVE (Gentle, act Interested, be Validating, and keep an Easy manner) technique. In your daily interactions, aim to be gentle, interested, validating, and maintaining an effortless composure. This could include practicing active listening, displaying empathy, and being more aware of your body language and tone of voice.

'Healing begins with the loving embrace of our wounded inner child.'

Pema Chodron

—

CONCLUSION

W e have now come to an end of the book. Within you, the wounded inner child now no longer needs to be an endless source of pain. While your physical form links you to the past, the passage of time has created a space for personal growth, healing, and triumph. You must remember that through overcoming adversity and navigating life's challenges, you have emerged as someone deserving of immense pride.

By utilizing the tools and exercises in this book, you have embarked on a journey of self-discovery and self-compassion. You have learned to understand the roots of your pain and navigate your emotions' complexities. With each passing week, you have gained insights, developed coping strategies, and embraced healing modalities that have empowered you to release the shackles of the past and step into a brighter, more authentic future.

I want to remind you that the benefits you have gained from this journey are not to be underestimated. You have not only gained a deeper understanding of yourself and your past, but also cultivated a greater sense of self-compassion and self-love. You have learned to hold your wounds with tenderness and to nurture the vulnerable parts of yourself that were once neglected. Through the delicate process of reparenting, you have offered solace, safety, and validation to your wounded inner child, allowing them to heal and flourish.

Remember that the healing journey is ongoing as you move forward from this transformative experience. It is not limited to a specific timeframe or confined to the pages of this book. It is a lifelong commitment to self-care, self-discovery, and self-love. Embrace the knowledge and tools you have gained, and carry them with you as guiding beacons in your daily life.

I want to emphasize that you are not alone on this journey. If you find that you need additional support or guidance, do not hesitate to seek professional help. The path to healing is unique for each individual, and there is strength in reaching out for assistance when needed. Surround yourself with a compassionate support system, and remember there is no shame in asking for help.

As you nurture your inner child and continue to grow, remember that you are celebrating the resilient spirit within you. You have come so far, defying the odds and transcending the pain of your past. You have reclaimed your voice, authenticity, and capacity to love and be loved.

By acknowledging and validating your inner child's needs, you have opened the door to a future filled with self-compassion, emotional expression, and a renewed sense of worthiness. Embrace the wisdom of your inner child, and allow their playful spirit to guide you as you navigate life's joys and challenges.

Know that you are enough. You are strong enough. You deserve the love, care, and healing you wholeheartedly deserve. The portal to healing your past remains open, offering you endless opportunities for growth and transformation.

You were strong enough to make it through your childhood with a good heart and determination to become whole; that's why you read this book. Go toward the future knowing you are good enough, you are strong enough, and you are worthy of the space you fill on this Earth with your unique perspective.

There is no portal in time that closes the opportunity for you to heal your past. Nurturing your inner child, acknowledging them, and validating their needs, will allow you to learn to express your emotions in a productive and healthy way while simultaneously learning to love the unique gift that you are.

Made in the USA
Las Vegas, NV
20 January 2025

16698735R10136